MONASH UNIVERSITY LOW FODMAP: THE COOKBOOK

THE MONASH FODMAP TEAM

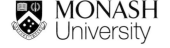

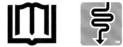

MONASH UNIVERSITY LOW FODMAP: THE COOKBOOK

Monash University Publishing
Matheson Library Annexe
40 Exhibition Walk
Monash University
Clayton, Victoria 3800, Australia
publishing.monash.edu

ISBN: 978-1-922633-30-9

A catalogue record for this book is available from the National Library of Australia.

Printed in Australia by Adams Print.

CONTENTS

INTRODUCTION

Monash University Low FODMAP: The Cookbook brings together fresh, nourishing, low FODMAP ingredients to create delicious, simple dishes from around the world. Inspired by our love of food and passion for enabling people to manage their IBS through diet, we hope this cookbook will make your FODMAP journey an enjoyable one.

This cookbook is the culmination of years of research focussed on improving the lives of people with medically diagnosed irritable bowel syndrome (IBS), using a diet therapy known as the FODMAP diet. IBS is an extremely common gut disorder affecting 1 in 7 adults and the FODMAP diet has revolutionised the treatment of this condition, providing symptom relief when previously there was none.
The FODMAP diet is an evidence-based therapy that restricts a group of short chain carbohydrates found in a wide range of foods and improves IBS symptoms in 3 out of 4 IBS sufferers.[1]
The diet involves swapping high FODMAP foods for low FODMAP alternatives and has helped millions of people from around the world to better manage their IBS symptoms.

Years of groundbreaking research enabled our team of dietitians, scientists and gastroenterologists to establish the effectiveness of this diet [1-3] and further our understanding of how FODMAPs trigger symptoms of IBS.[4-5] We also tested the FODMAP content of hundreds of foods sourced from all over the world.[6-8] And to enable people worldwide to follow this diet, we developed the Monash University FODMAP Diet App. This App provides quick and easy access to information regarding the FODMAP content of all laboratory tested by our team for FODMAP content.

INTRODUCING THE MONASH UNIVERSITY LOW FODMAP STACK CUP

We have long recognised that single foods do not make a diet. People eat combinations of foods and whole meals and want to know that each recipe, and indeed each combination of recipes, is low in FODMAPs. To make this possible, this cookbook introduces the new Monash University Low FODMAP Stack Cup. Using the Monash University Low FODMAP Stack Cup, one full cup represents the upper limit of FODMAPs that most people will tolerate in one sitting. Using this symbol, you can mix and match recipes from this cookbook to create delicious, low FODMAP meal plans. Be it walnut, seed and coconut granola for breakfast and salad Nicoise for lunch or lasagne for dinner, the Monash University Low FODMAP Stack Cup allows you to quickly and easily understand what you can eat in one sitting, without triggering IBS symptoms.

Not only are recipes in this cookbook packed full of flavour, they're also nutritious. We know that without careful planning, a low FODMAP diet can compromise intake of several key nutrients. To address this, we've included nutrient symbols, so you can quickly identify dishes that are good sources of iron (Fe), calcium (Ca), protein (Pr) and dietary fibre (DF), and we've enabled people following gluten free (GF), vegan (Ve) and/or vegetarian (V) diets to find suitable recipes.

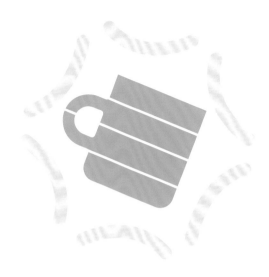

THE MONASH FODMAP TEAM

The research team at Monash University are the founders of the FODMAP diet.[1,4,5,9] Our team introduced the FODMAP concept and developed the first FODMAP diet. We conducted the first studies to show that a low FODMAP diet reduces symptoms in 75% of people with IBS;[1] demonstrated the mechanisms by which FODMAPs trigger gut symptoms[4,5] and built a large database describing the FODMAP composition of food.[6-8,10] Findings from our research have since been replicated by dozens of research groups around the world, and the real-world experience of patients using this diet has been overwhelmingly positive. This evidence is now reflected in clinical guidelines and practice, whereby a low FODMAP diet is recommended as a first-line IBS treatment in Australia, the UK, the USA, Canada, Japan and Korea. The low FODMAP diet has helped millions of people with IBS worldwide to manage their symptoms and improve their quality of life using this evidence-based diet.

BEGINNING A LOW FODMAP DIET

WHAT IS IBS?

IBS is a very common gastrointestinal disorder that affects around 1 in 7 people. People with IBS usually experience abdominal (tummy) pain and abnormal bowel habits (such as diarrhoea, constipation, or a combination of both). Other common symptoms include bloating, distension and excessive flatulence (wind or gas).

Certain sugars found in foods are known to trigger symptoms of IBS and these sugars are known as FODMAPs. FODMAP is an acronym which stands for Fermentable Oligosaccharides, Disaccharides, Monosaccharides, And Polyols.

FODMAPs are found in many commonly consumed foods, including fruit and vegetables, grains and cereals, nuts, legumes, dairy foods and manufactured foods. Most people eat FODMAPs in their every day diet without problems, but people with IBS have a highly sensitive gut wall. In people with IBS, FODMAPs can trigger gastrointestinal symptoms, including pain, excessive flatulence, bloating, distension and abnormal bowel habit.

F ermentable
O ligosaccharides
D isaccharides
M onosaccharides
A nd
P olyols

WHAT IS A FODMAP DIET?

A FODMAP diet is a 3 step diet. It is important you follow all 3 steps of the FODMAP diet as this will help you to understand whether your IBS symptoms are sensitive to FODMAPs. Step 1 of the FODMAP Diet will help you to understand whether you are among the 3 in 4 IBS sufferers who improve on the diet, or the 1 in 4 sufferers who do not. If your symptoms do not improve on a low FODMAP diet, you may need to consider other IBS therapies. The 3 steps will also help you determine which foods and FODMAPs you tolerate, and which trigger your IBS symptoms. Understanding this will help you to personalise your FODMAP diet and follow a less restrictive, more nutritionally balanced diet for the long term that only restricts foods that trigger your IBS symptoms. This cookbook is particularly useful in Step 1 of the FODMAP diet, as all the recipes are low in FODMAPs.

CONFIRM YOUR DIAGNOSIS

If you suspect you have IBS, see your medical doctor for a proper diagnosis. Do not self-diagnose. Your doctor can run tests to rule out other conditions such as coeliac disease, inflammatory bowel disease and endometriosis. Once you are diagnosed with IBS, you can choose treatments that are best targeted to your condition.

STEP 1.
LOW FODMAP
(2–6 WEEKS)

THE AIM OF STEP 1 IS TO IMPROVE IBS SYMPTOMS.

Foods that are **high** and **moderate** in FODMAPs are swapped for **low** FODMAP alternatives. For example, pears (a high FODMAP fruit) might be swapped for kiwi fruit (a low FODMAP fruit). Step 1 should be followed for around 2 to 6 weeks.

Use the Food Guide of the Monash University FODMAP Diet App to identify high (red), moderate (amber) and low (green) FODMAP foods.

You will eat mostly low FODMAP foods in this step.

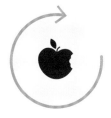

STEP 2.
REINTRODUCTION

THE AIM OF STEP 2 IS TO IDENTIFY WHICH FODMAPS YOU TOLERATE AND WHICH TRIGGER YOUR IBS SYMPTOMS.

In this step, you continue your **low FODMAP diet.**
At the same time you will complete a series of food challenges to help you understand which foods and FODMAPs you tolerate and which trigger your symptoms.

The diary function of the Monash University FODMAP Diet App will help you to identify suitable challenge foods and to record symptom responses to each challenge.

STEP 3.
PERSONALISATION

THE AIM OF STEP 3 IS TO RELAX DIETARY RESTRICTIONS, EXPAND YOUR DIET AND ESTABLISH A 'PERSONALISED FODMAP DIET' FOR THE LONG-TERM.

By now you should understand which FODMAPs you tolerate and which trigger your symptoms.

Foods and FODMAPs that are well tolerated are included in your diet, while poorly tolerated foods and FODMAPs are restricted, but only to a level needed to maintain symptom relief.

The filters in the Monash University FODMAP Diet App can be used to tailor the Food Guide to suit your personal FODMAP sensitivities.

Over time, continue to challenge poorly tolerated, higher FODMAP foods as your tolerance can change.

THE MONASH UNIVERSITY FODMAP DIET APP

The Monash University FODMAP Diet App provides easy access to information about the FODMAP content of foods. All foods included in the App have been laboratory tested by the Monash FODMAP team for FODMAP content. A traffic light rating system is used to indicate which foods are low, moderate or high in FODMAPs.

The App is available for Android and iOS devices and can be downloaded from the the App Store, Google Play or the Amazon App Store. Revenue generated from App sales helps to fund further FODMAP food analysis and research.

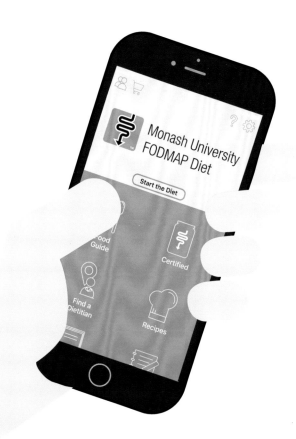

TIPS ON GETTING STARTED

- Plan your low FODMAP meals and snacks.
- Write a shopping list of low FODMAP fresh and staple foods.
- Consider whether you can adapt your existing recipes to make them low FODMAP.
- Be patient with yourself and give yourself time to get it right.
- See a Monash FODMAP trained dietitian for expert advice on IBS and the FODMAP diet.

WORKING WITH A DIETITIAN

The FODMAP diet is a therapeutic diet for IBS and should be trialled under the guidance of an experienced dietitian. A dietitian can help you to:

- work through the 3 steps of the diet
- plan your shopping list and meals
- design a nutritionally balanced, low FODMAP diet
- troubleshoot if your symptoms do not improve on the diet
- identify other therapies or health professionals that may help to relieve your IBS symptoms

Find Monash FODMAP trained dietitians on the Monash FODMAP Dietitian Directory (monashfodmap.com/online-training/fodmap-dietitians-directory).

NUTRITIONAL ADVICE

A low FODMAP diet involves restricting certain foods from your diet, so careful planning is needed to ensure it is nutritionally balanced.

For example, dairy foods (which are rich sources of calcium) are also high in lactose and therefore restricted on a low FODMAP diet. But instead of eliminating dairy foods from your diet, we recommend you SWAP high FODMAP dairy foods in your diet for low FODMAP dairy alternatives. For example, instead of drinking cow's milk, drink lactose-free cow's milk or a low FODMAP milk alternative, such as almond milk or soy milk (made from soy protein). If using milk alternatives, look for calcium fortified varieties.

The Monash University FODMAP Diet App will help you to identify high FODMAP foods in your diet and suitable low FODMAP alternatives.

When planning your low FODMAP diet, try to include adequate serves of foods from each of the 5 food groups. Examples of high and low FODMAP foods from each of the food groups are included in the table below (see page 16).

HOW TO USE THIS BOOK

MONASH UNIVERSITY LOW FODMAP STACK CUP

The Monash University Low FODMAP stack symbol can be used to mix and match dishes and plan your low FODMAP meals. The symbol indicates the amount of FODMAPs provided in one serve of each dish, relative to the amount you should tolerate in one sitting.

We know that most people tolerate 0.5 grams of FODMAPs in one sitting. Using our stacking symbol, each band represents 0.125 grams of FODMAPs (or ¼ of your FODMAP limit per meal). This means that you can include up to 4 bands per meal, before you 'fill your cup' and reach your 0.5 grams FODMAP limit for that meal.[11]

For example, at dinner you may want to eat 1 serve of the French lamb shanks (1 band), 1 serve of the roasted vegetables with balsamic (3 bands). This would provide 4 bands in total, meaning you have reached your FODMAP limit for that meal.

After 2–3 hours, we assume that the 'cup' returns to zero.

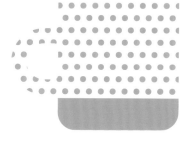

The **'low FODMAP stack one'** symbol indicates that you can add more FODMAP-containing foods (no more than 3 bands) to your meal.

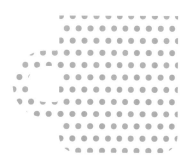

The **'low FODMAP stack zero'** symbol indicates a meal that contains trace amounts of FODMAPs.

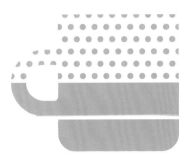

The 'low FODMAP stack two' symbol indicates that you can add more FODMAP-containing foods (no more than 2 bands) to your meal.

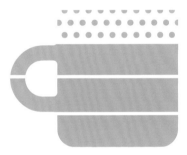

The 'low FODMAP stack three' symbol indicates that you can add more FODMAP-containing foods (no more than 1 band) to your meal.

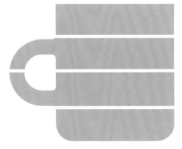

The 'low FODMAP stack four' symbol indicates that you have reached the low FODMAP limit. To ensure that your meal is low FODMAP do not add any additional FODMAP-containing foods to this meal.

NUTRIENT SYMBOLS

This cookbook includes icons to indicate whether each dish is a
good source of protein, calcium, iron and/or fibre.
We have focussed on these nutrients because we know that they
can be lacking in a low FODMAP diet.[12] Recipes marked with any
one of these symbols meet criteria set by Food Standards Australia
New Zealand (FSANZ).[13]

VEGETARIAN

There are several types of vegetarian diets, including
lacto-vegetarian (which includes dairy foods), ovo-lacto (which
includes dairy foods and eggs) and vegan (which includes only plant
foods). In this book, the vegetarian symbol indicates ovo-lacto
vegetarian dishes that do not include any meat, poultry or seafood,
but do include dairy foods (such as cheese), eggs and plant foods.

VEGAN

The vegan symbol indicates dishes that include only plant-based
foods, and exclude meat, poultry, seafood, dairy products, eggs,
honey and other animal-derived ingredients, such as oyster sauce,
fish sauce and gelatine.

GLUTEN-FREE

Dishes marked with this symbol are gluten free. Gluten is a protein found in wheat, rye,
oats and barley. Although gluten restriction is not necessary to manage the symptoms
of irritable bowel syndrome, for people who have coeliac disease, a strict, life-long
gluten-free diet is the only form of treatment. We have included the gluten-free symbol in
this book because we acknowledge that a large proportion of consumers are following a
gluten-free diet (often unnecessarily) and thus looking for gluten-free recipes.

PROTEIN

Recipes with the protein symbol contain at least **10g of protein per
serve.** Protein is essential for our cells to grow and repair, and to
build strong muscles and healthy bones. Protein is especially
important for people following vegan or vegetarian diets as many
plant-based, protein rich foods are also high in FODMAPs and
restricted on a low FODMAP diet.

Recommended daily intake −[14]
46g/day (women 19–70 years)
64g/day (men 19–70 years)

CALCIUM

Dishes carrying the calcium symbol provide **at least 200mg calcium per serve.** Calcium is essential for strong bones and healthy teeth, and dairy foods are the richest natural sources of calcium. However, because some dairy foods are high in lactose, intake of dairy foods and calcium can be inadequate on a low FODMAP diet.

Recommended daily intake –[14]
1000 mg/day (women 19–50 years, men 19–70 years)
1300mg/day (women >50 years, men >70 years)

IRON

The iron symbol indicates dishes that contain **at least 4.5mg of iron per serve.** Iron is essential for red blood cell production, the transport of oxygen around the body, a healthy immune system and for releasing energy from cells. Iron intake can be inadequate on a low FODMAP diet because many plant-based, iron-rich foods (such as wholegrain breads and cereals, nuts and dried fruits) are also high in FODMAPs and restricted on the diet. Women typically need more iron than men, so our cut off for the iron symbol was set conservatively and represents 25% of the recommended daily intake (RDI) for iron in women.

Recommended daily intake –[14]
18mg/day (women 19–50 years)
8mg/day (men >18 years, women >50 years)

DIETARY FIBRE

The fibre symbol indicates dishes that contain **at least 4g fibre per serve.** Fibre is essential for a healthy digestive system and a high fibre diet reduces our risk of conditions such as constipation, diverticular disease, bowel cancer and cardio-vascular disease. Fibre intake can be compromised on a low FODMAP diet because many high fibre foods (such as fruits, vegetables, grains, cereals, nuts and legumes) are also high in FODMAPs and thus restricted on the diet.

Recommended daily intake –[14]
25g/day (women >18 years)
30g/day (men >18 years)

VEGAN AND VEGETARIAN NUTRIENT SOURCES

While vegetarian and vegan diets can be very healthy and reduce the risk of a number of chronic diseases, careful planning is needed to ensure they are nutritionally adequate, especially in people adhering to other dietary restrictions, such as a low FODMAP diet.[10]

Nutrients at risk on a vegetarian, low FODMAP diet include protein, iron, zinc, and B12. Intake of these nutrients can also be compromised on a vegan diet, as can intake of calcium and omega 3 fatty acids.

The following table describes low FODMAP, vegetarian and vegan foods that are rich in these nutrients.[15]

LOW FODMAP PLANT-BASED SOURCES OF IMPORTANT NUTRIENTS

Suitable for both vegan and vegetarian diets

CALCIUM	PROTEIN
▪ Fortified plant-based milks, cheeses and yoghurts (macadamia milk, soy milk made from soy protein, almond milk, rice milk, soy cheese, coconut yoghurt) ▪ Soy products (firm tofu, tempeh) ▪ Nuts (almonds) ▪ Seeds (sesame seeds, poppy seeds) ▪ Green leafy vegetables (kale, spinach, bok choy)	▪ Pulses (canned chickpeas, canned lentils) ▪ Nuts (almonds, walnuts, peanuts, macadamias) ▪ Soy products (firm tofu, soy milk made from soy protein, tempeh) ▪ Seeds (sesame, chia, poppy, pumpkin, sunflower, linseeds) ▪ Spreads (tahini, peanut butter)

LOW FODMAP ANIMAL-BASED SOURCES OF IMPORTANT NUTRIENTS

Suitable for vegetarian diets

CALCIUM	PROTEIN
▪ Dairy sources (cheddar cheese, low-lactose cow's milk, low-lactose yoghurt)	▪ Dairy sources (cheddar cheese, low-lactose cow's milk, low-lactose yoghurt) ▪ Eggs

ZINC	VITAMIN B12	OMEGA 3 FATTY ACIDS	IRON
• Pulses (canned chickpeas, canned lentils) • Soy products (firm tofu, tempeh) • Nuts (pecans, peanuts, brazil nuts, pine nuts, almonds, walnuts) • Seeds (chia seeds, pumpkin seeds, sesame seeds, sunflower seeds, poppy seeds) • Spreads (tahini, yeast extracts)	• Fortified plant-based milk alternatives (macadamia milk, soy milk made from soy protein, almond milk, rice milk, oat milk)	• Seeds (flax seeds, chia seeds, hemp seeds) • Nuts (walnuts) • Plant-based oils (Flaxseed oil, soybean oil, canola oil, chia oil, walnut oil, hemp seed oil)	• Pulses (canned chickpeas, canned lentils, edamame) • Nuts (almond, pine nuts, peanuts) • Grains (oats, quinoa) • Spreads (almond butter, tahini) • Seeds (chia seeds, flax seeds, pumpkin seeds, hemp seeds, sesame seeds, sunflower seeds) • Soy products (firm tofu, tempeh) • Potato (sweet potato) • Green leafy vegetables (kale, broccoli, broccolini, spinach, bok choy)

ZINC	VITAMIN B12	OMEGA 3 FATTY ACIDS	IRON
• Dairy sources (cheddar cheese, low-lactose cow's milk, low-lactose yoghurt)	• Dairy sources (cheddar cheese, low-lactose cow's milk, low-lactose yoghurt) • Eggs	• Eggs	• Eggs

HEALTHY EATING ON A LOW FODMAP DIET

To ensure that your diet is nutritionally balanced while following a low FODMAP diet eat a variety of foods from each of the six main food groups.

This infographic shows how much food from each food group needs to be consumed every day.[16] Simply swap high FODMAP foods (shown in red) with low FODMAP alternatives (shown in green).

FRUIT (2 SERVES)

PEAR
1 MED

APPLE
1 MED

VEGETABLES (5–7 SERVES)

SAVOY CABBAGE
½ CUP

CAULIFLOWER
½ CUP

ASPARAGUS
½ CUP

BUTTON MUSHROOMS
½ CUP

PEAS
½ CUP

DAIRY (2–4 SERVES)

CHEESE
40g

FULL CREAM MILK
1 CUP

FATS (LIMIT)

OIL
LIMIT SERVES

PROTEIN (2–3 SERVES)

CHICKPEAS/RED
KIDNEY BEANS
CANNED OR COOKED
1 CUP 150g

RED MEAT
65g COOKED

EGGS
2 EGGS

BREAD, CEREALS, PASTA AND NOODLES (4–6 SERVES)

MUESLI
¼ CUP

COUS COUS
½ CUP

WHEAT PASTA
1 CUP

MULTIGRAIN BREAD
2 SLICES

* — these foods are good sources of protein and/or fats and do not contain any FODMAPs

FRUIT (2 SERVES)

 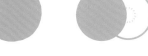

ORANGE
1 MED

KIWI FRUIT
1 MED

VEGETABLES (5–7 SERVES)

GREEN BEANS
½ CUP

POTATO
½ 1 MED

GREEN CAPSICUM
½ CUP

CARROT
½ CUP

EGGPLANT
½ CUP

DAIRY (2–4 SERVES)

FATS (LIMIT)

PROTEIN (2–3 SERVES)

HARD CHEESE/
LOW LACTOSE
SOFT CHEESE
40g

LACTOSE FREE MILK
1 CUP

OIL
LIMIT SERVES

FIRM TOFU
170g

RED MEAT
65g COOKED

EGGS
2 EGGS

BREAD, CEREALS, PASTA AND NOODLES (4–6 SERVES)

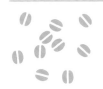

ROLLED OATS
½ CUP

BROWN RICE
½ CUP

GLUTEN FREE PASTA
1 CUP

SOURDOUGH
SPELT BREAD
2 SLICES

LOW FODMAP PANTRY

Below is a list of low FODMAP foods that are used throughout the cookbook.
In some recipes we have been quite specific with the types of ingredients to use, this is because we have selected the ingredient with the lowest FODMAP content.

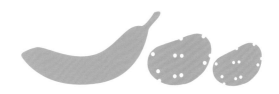

VEGETABLES

- Green capsicum (bell pepper)* —these have the lowest levels of FODMAPs compared to red and yellow varieties.

- Red capsicum (bell pepper)* — higher in FODMAPs than green and yellow varieties. Use the serve size specified in the recipe.

- Spring onion (scallion) green tops only — use the green tops only as the bulb is high in FODMAPs.

- Leek greens (green tops only) — Use the green tops only as the bulb is high in FODMAPs.

- Chilli* — a variety can be used (refer to the Monash FODMAP app).

- Tomatoes (common/truss) — these varieties have the lowest levels of FODMAPs.

- Cherry tomatoes — these variety of tomatoes are higher in FODMAPs. Use the serve size given in the recipes.

- Tinned whole tomatoes (Roma/Plum) — this type of tinned tomatoes contains the lowest levels of FODMAPs.

- Chinese broccoli

- Cabbage, wombok

- Kent pumpkin (squash)

- Cucumber — lebanese or common

- Potato — common types may be used

- Oyster mushroom — oyster mushrooms are low in the FODMAP-mannitol.

FRUIT

- Banana (firm) — firm bananas lowest in FODMAPs are yellow with a greenish tinge.

BREADS AND CEREALS

Look for Monash University low FODMAP certified brands

- Low FODMAP sourdough bread/low FODMAP bread — traditional sourdough breads (particularly sourdough spelt bread) are naturally lower in FODMAPs. Gluten-free breads can also be lower in FODMAPs (check that the bread is made with low FODMAP ingredients e.g. rice flour, corn flour/starch, maize flour, tapioca flour/starch, potato flour/starch). Look out for Monash low FODMAP certified breads.

- Rice, brown or white, medium grain, short or long grain

- Rice noodles — all, soba noodles

- Oats

- Quinoa

- Polenta, instant polenta

- Pasta/spaghetti — Many commercially available gluten free pastas/spaghetti made with low FODMAP ingredients (e.g. rice flour, corn flour/starch, maize flour, tapioca flour/starch, potato flour/starch) are suitable however always check the ingredient list for potentially high FODMAP ingredients (such as chickpea flour, soy flour and lupin flour).

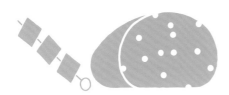

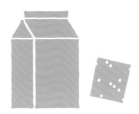

FLOURS

- Gluten-free flour/low FODMAP flour. Many commercially available gluten free flours made with low FODMAP ingredients (e.g. rice flour, corn flour/starch, maize flour, tapioca flour/starch, potato flour/starch) are suitable however always check the ingredient list for potentially high FODMAP ingredients (such as chickpea flour, soy flour and lupin flour).

PULSES/VEGETARIAN SUBSTITUTES

- Canned lentils, drained rinsed
- Canned chickpeas, drained rinsed
- Firm tofu — do not use silken

DAIRY/DAIRY SUBSTITUTES

- Lactose-free milk
- Lactose-free yoghurt
- Lactose-free Greek yoghurt — see recipes in the 'basics' section of the cookbook.
- Lactose-free cream
- Soy milk (made from soy protein) calcium-fortified
- Almond milk (calcium-fortified)
- Cheese — pecorino, parmesan, paneer and cheddar cheese (use the serve size given in recipes).

NUTS/SEEDS

- Tahini, hulled or unhulled
- Nuts — walnut, pine nut, peanuts all specified as low FODMAP
- Seeds — sesame, poppy, hemp, linseeds/flaxseeds, chia seeds, pepitas

OIL

- Garlic-infused olive oil

STOCKS

- Stocks — chicken, vegetable and beef
- See recipes in the 'basics' section of the cookbook and look for Monash University low FODMAP certified brands.

* — Please note that capsicum (bell pepper) and chilli also contain capsaicin, a natural ingredient which gives a spicy flavor and can trigger heartburn and abdominal pain in some individuals with IBS.

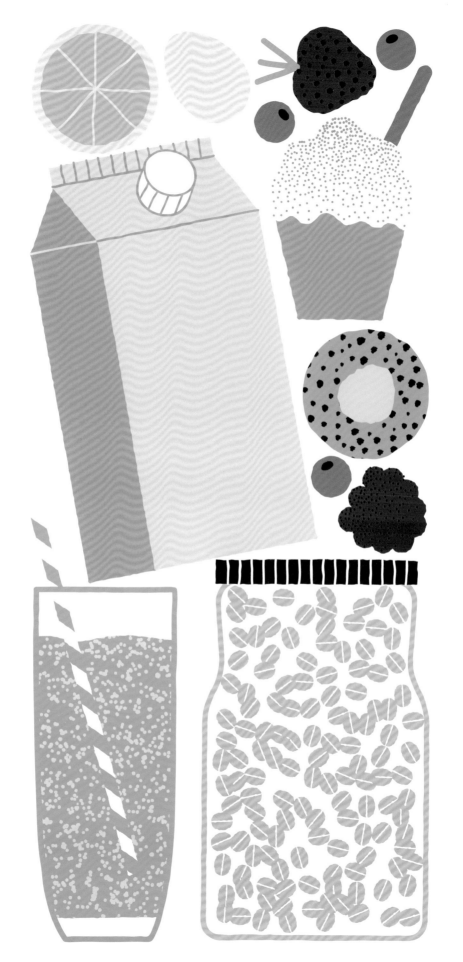

BREAKFAST

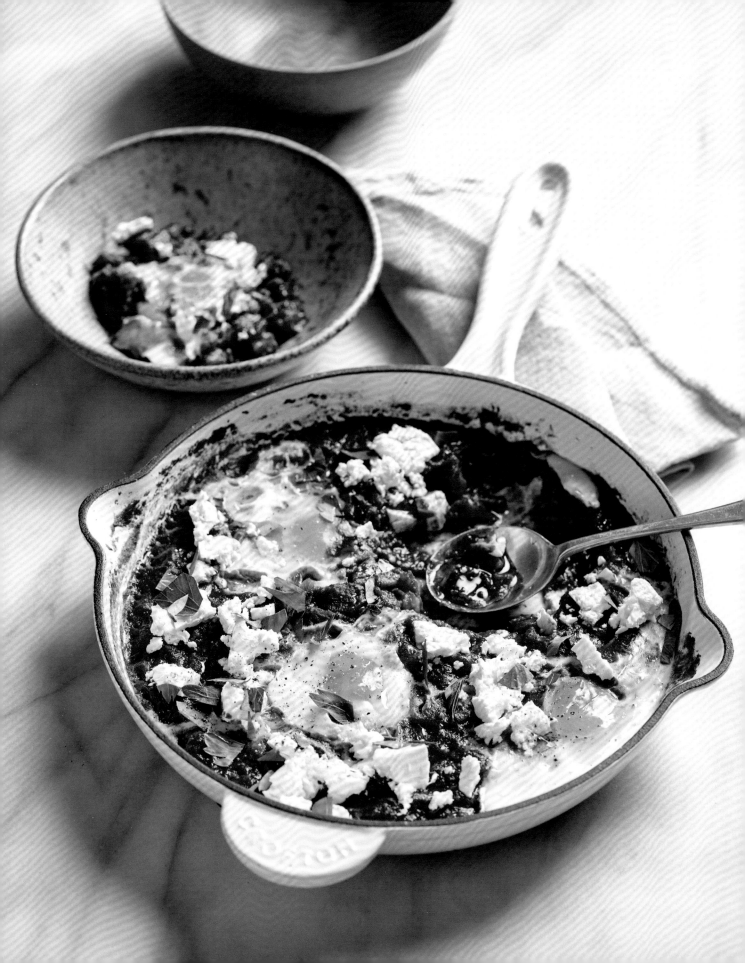

SHAKSHOUKA

SERVES 4

3 tbsp garlic-infused olive oil

half a medium-sized eggplant
  (aubergine), diced

1 green capsicum (bell pepper),
  deseeded and diced

1 tsp paprika

¼ tsp black pepper

½ tsp cumin

800g (1lb 8oz) tinned whole
  tomatoes, chopped

¼ cup water

4 eggs

100g (3½oz) fetta

¼ cup parsley, roughly chopped

salt to taste

Energy 1316kJ/314 Calories, Protein
13.4g, Total Fat 23.5g, Saturated Fat 6.7g,
Carbohydrate 9.4g, Sugars 9.3g, Dietary
fibre 5.0g, Calcium 168.5mg, Iron 3.4mg.

1. Heat the garlic-infused olive oil in a large pan over medium heat. Add the eggplant and capsicum and sauté for 5 minutes or until softened slightly.

2. Reduce the heat and add all of the spices. Cook for 1 minute, stirring constantly until fragrant.

3. Add the tinned tomato, bring to the boil and then reduce the heat to medium-low. Pour the water around the tomato tins and swirl around to get all of the excess tomato from the tins. Add the water to the pan to loosen the mixture – you may not need all of it. Cook for 20-25 mins or until thickened.

4. Remove the pan from the heat once the mixture has thickened. Create hollows in the sauce for each of the eggs and carefully break an egg into each hollow.

5. Place the pan back on the heat and cover with a lid. Cook for an additional 7-8 minutes or until the eggs have cooked through.

6. Remove from heat and garnish with fetta and parsley.

CARROT AND ZUCCHINI FRITTERS WITH POACHED EGGS

SERVES 4 (MAKES 12)

3 medium-sized carrots, grated

170g (6oz) zucchini (courgette), grated

½ cup gluten-free flour

1 tsp ground cumin

1 tsp ground coriander

½ cup coriander leaves (cilantro),
   roughly chopped

½ cup spring onions (scallions) (green
   tops only), roughly chopped

1 egg, whisked

½ tsp sea salt

pepper to taste

2 tbsp garlic-infused olive oil

4 eggs, poached

Energy 1157kJ/276 Calories, Protein
10.2g, Total Fat 15.2g, Saturated Fat 2.9g,
Carbohydrate 22.7g, Sugars 7.7g, Dietary
fibre 4.5g, Calcium 82.1mg, Iron 2.9mg.

1. Place the carrot and zucchini in a sieve. Using a paper towel, press into the sieve to draw out the excess moisture.

2. In a large bowl, combine the carrot, zucchini (courgette), gluten-free flour, spices, coriander (cilantro), spring onion tops (scallions), whisked egg and salt. Season with pepper and mix well until combined.

3. Heat 1 tbsp of garlic-infused olive oil in a large fry pan over medium heat. Scoop ¼ cup measurements of mixture into the pan and fry for approximately 3 minutes on each side. This will need to be done in batches.

4. Once the fritters are cooked, place them on a plate lined with paper towel to absorb any excess oil.

5. To serve, place the fritters on a plate and top each serve with a poached egg.

SERVING SUGGESTION

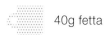 40g fetta

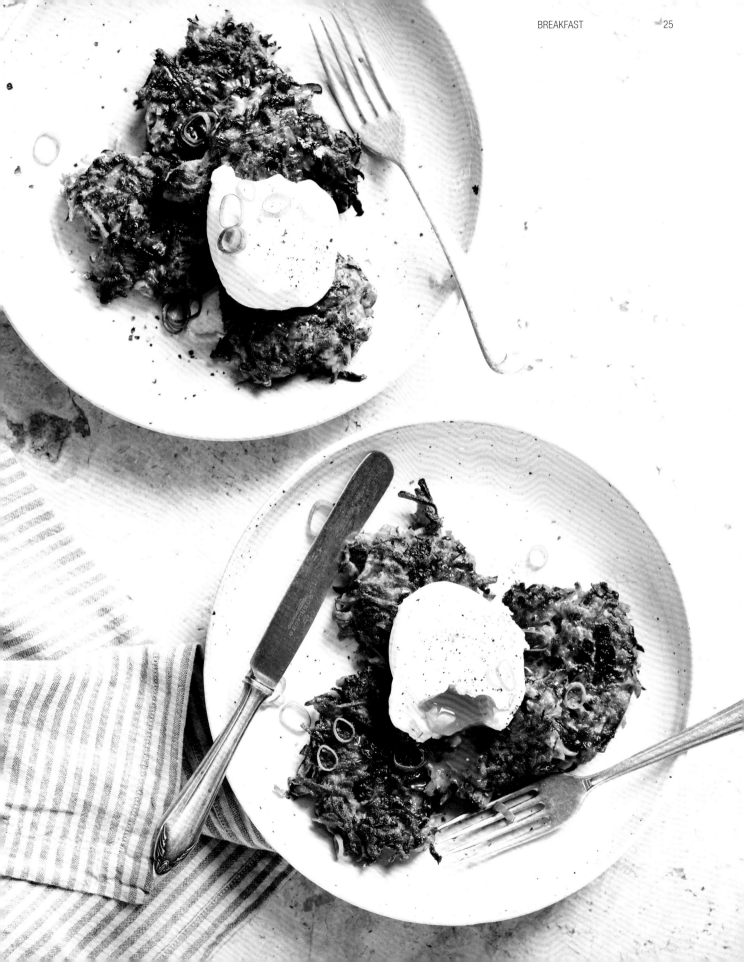

SPINACH, FETTA AND PINE NUT OMELETTE

    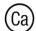

SERVES 1

1 cup baby spinach leaves,
   firmly packed
¼ cup fetta, crumbled
2 large eggs
1 tbsp lactose-free milk
ground black pepper to taste
5g (1 tsp) butter
1 tbsp pine nuts

Energy 1638 kJ/391 Calories, Protein
24.9g, Total Fat 31.6g, Saturated Fat 10.0g,
Carbohydrate 2.3g, Sugars 1.9g, Dietary
fibre 1.8g, Calcium 225.0mg, Iron 3.6 mg.

1. Wilt the spinach leaves in a lightly oiled pan over medium-low heat and fold through the fetta. Set aside.

2. Lightly whisk the eggs with milk and a pinch of pepper.

3. Preheat a non-stick fry pan over medium heat and add the butter. Spread the butter over the surface of the pan until it starts to sizzle.

4. Pour the egg and milk mixture into the frypan and swirl the pan to create a round omelette shape. Cover with a tightly fitting lid and cook until the omelette is almost cooked.

5. Spoon the spinach filling over half the omelette, cover and cook for approximately 20 seconds. Remove the lid and sprinkle with pine nuts.

6. Tip the pan towards the serving plate and fold the omelette in half to encase the filling.

7. Slide the cooked omelette onto the plate and serve with low FODMAP toast.

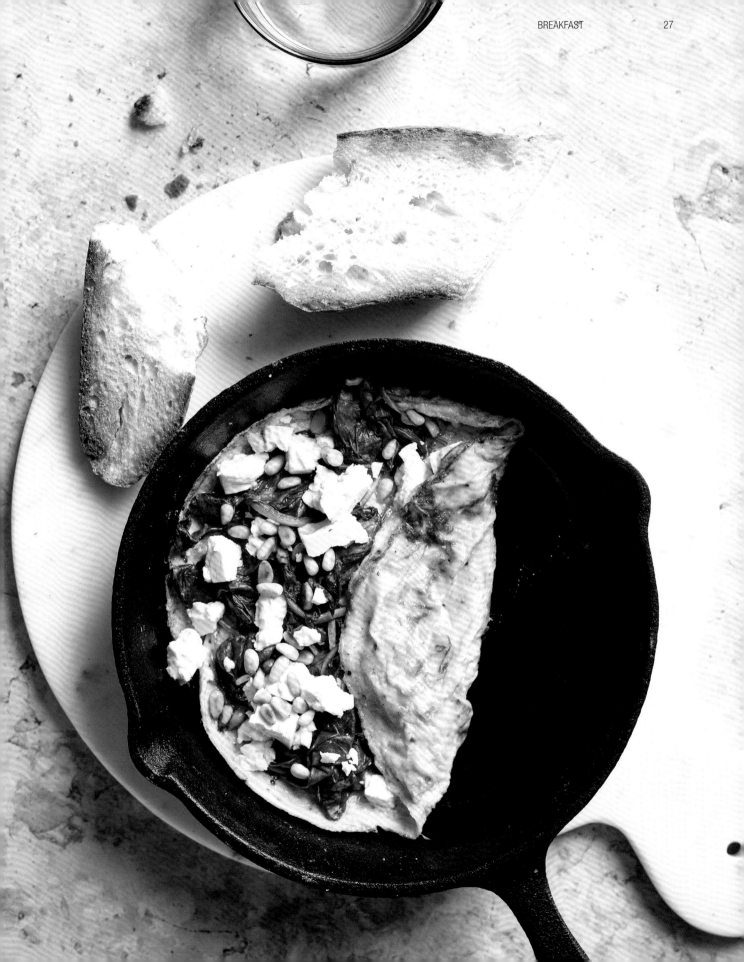

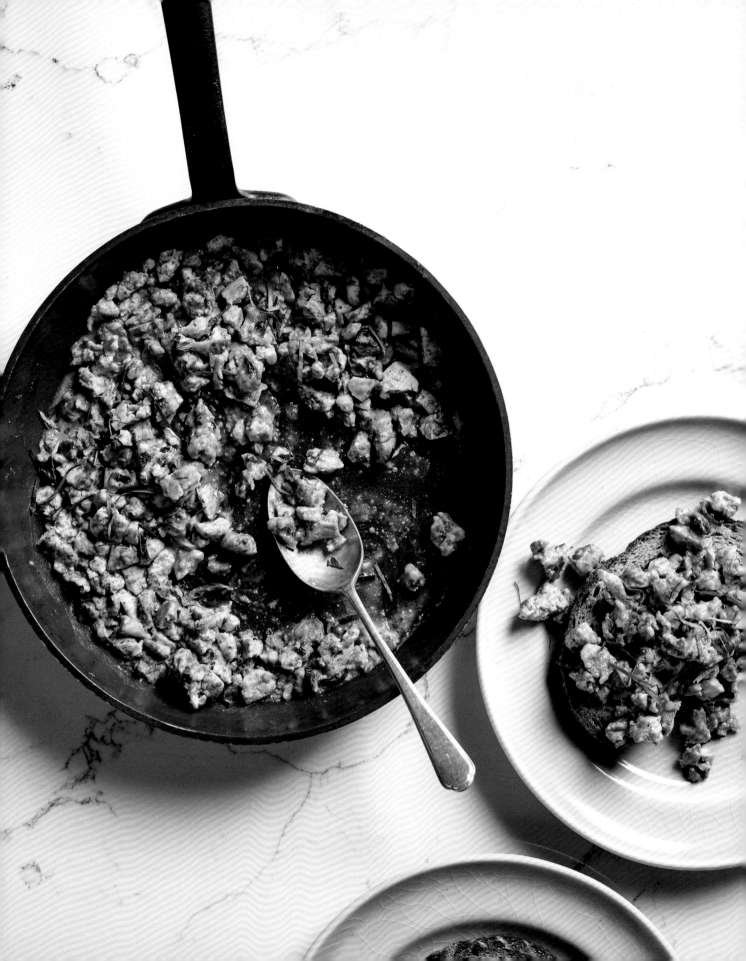

SCRAMBLED TOFU

SERVES 2

SCRAMBLE SAUCE
1 tbsp cornflour (cornstarch)
½ tsp turmeric
½ tsp paprika
1 tsp Dijon mustard
¼ tsp black pepper
½ cup soy milk
salt to taste

SCRAMBLE
250g (9oz) firm tofu
1 tbsp garlic-infused olive oil
½ cup spring onions (scallions) (green
    tops only), finely chopped
½ cup parsley, finely chopped
2 slices low FODMAP sourdough bread

Energy 1515 kJ/362 Calories, Protein
20.4g, Total Fat 21.0g, Saturated Fat 3.0g,
Carbohydrate 19.6g, Sugars 2.4g, Dietary
fibre 6.9g, Calcium 444.3mg, Iron 5.5mg.

1. To make the sauce, in a small saucepan, combine the cornflour (cornstarch), turmeric, paprika, Dijon mustard and black pepper. Gradually whisk in the soy milk.

2. Stir the sauce over medium heat for approximately 2 minutes or until the sauce begins to thicken. Remove the sauce from the heat and set it aside.

3. To make the scramble, dry the firm tofu on absorbent paper towel and gently crumble with your hands.

4. Preheat a frypan over medium heat and add the oil. When hot, add the spring onion tops (scallion). Reduce the heat to low and sauté for 2-3 minutes. Add the crumbled tofu and fry until the tofu has browned.

5. Gently stir through the pre-prepared, sauce ensuring it is evenly mixed through the scramble. Sprinkle with parsley and serve with low FODMAP toast.

VEGAN FRENCH TOAST

SERVES 2

70g (2½oz) firm tofu

¼ cup low FODMAP soy milk (made from soy protein)

½ tsp vanilla essence (extract)

⅛ tsp cinnamon

2 slices of low FODMAP bread (sourdough is preferable)

1 tsp oil

maple syrup to serve

Energy 1651kJ/395 Calories, Protein 18.4g, Total Fat 9.3g, Saturated Fat 1.3g, Carbohydrate 54.5g, Sugars 18.1g, Dietary fibre 5.3g, Calcium 353.8mg, Iron 3.5mg.

1. Add the firm tofu, soy milk, vanilla and cinnamon to a blender and blitz until combined. If you do not have a blender, use a whisk and a small bowl.

2. Pour the tofu mixture into a shallow dish and add the bread.

3. Soak the bread for 1 minute, then flip it over and soak the other side.

4. Preheat a non-stick frypan over medium-high heat and add the oil or butter. When the oil or butter is hot, add the bread and fry until golden on one side, then flip it and cook the other side.

5. Serve immediately with maple syrup.

SERVING SUGGESTION

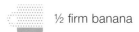 ½ firm banana

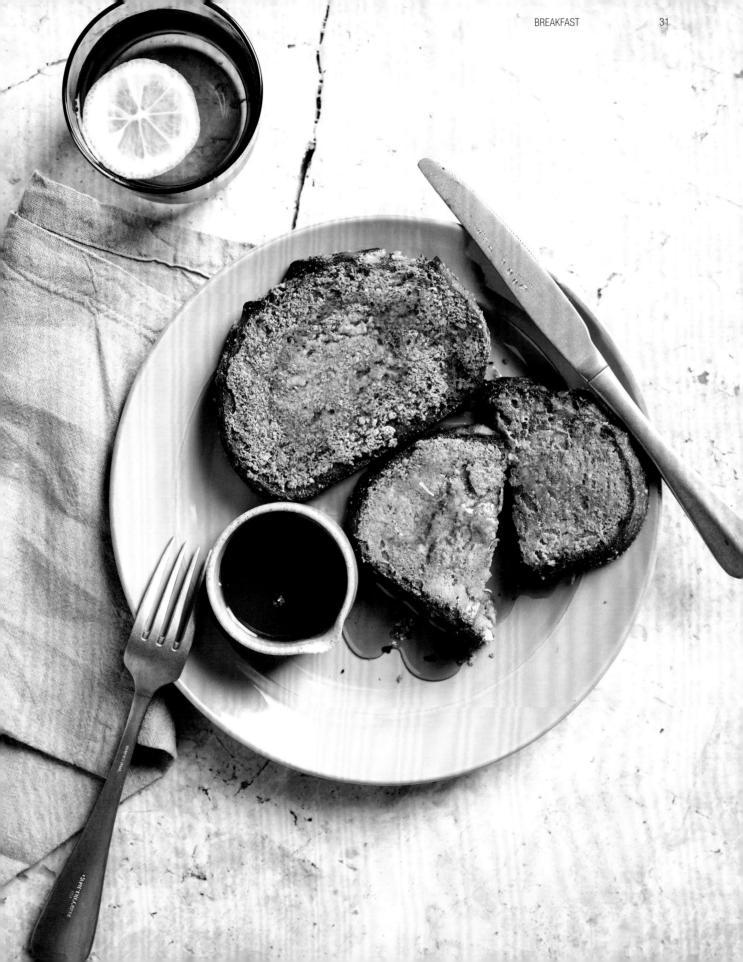

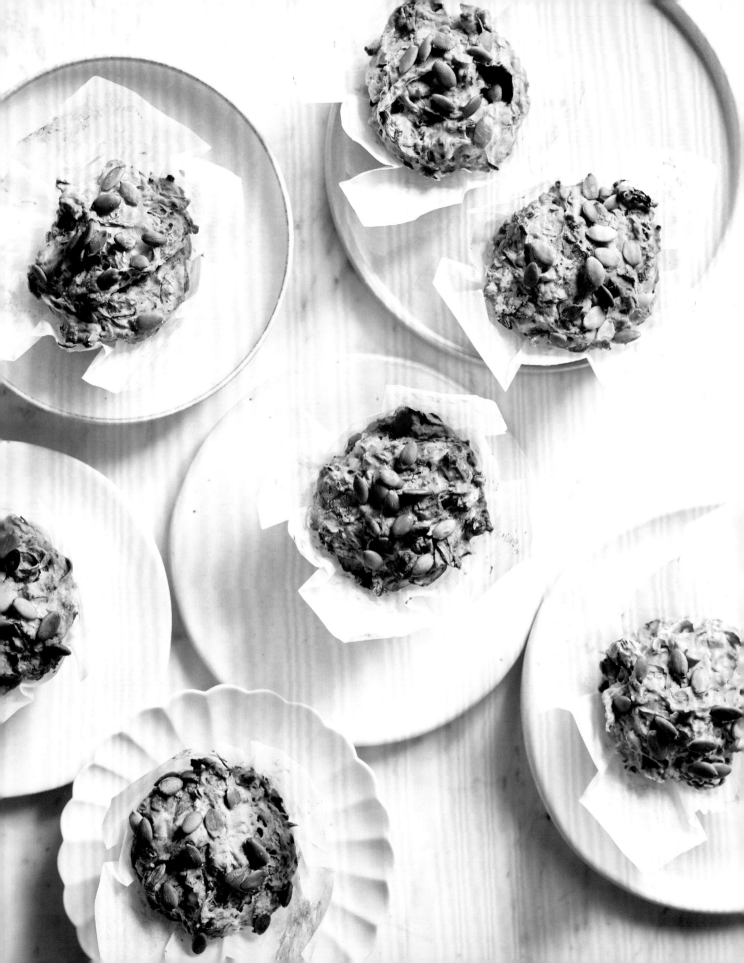

BREAKFAST MUFFINS

SERVES 9

2 cups gluten-free flour

2 tsp baking powder

2 cups grated kent pumpkin (squash)

60g (2oz) baby spinach, finely chopped

100g (3½oz) fetta, grated or crumbled

2 tsp smoked paprika

2 tbsp rosemary, finely chopped

1 egg, whisked

80g (3oz) butter, melted

1 cup lactose-free milk

2 tbsp pepitas

Energy 1048 kJ/250 Calories, Protein
6.1g, Total Fat 11.9g, Saturated Fat 5.3g,
Carbohydrate 28.8g, Sugars 2.9g, Dietary
fibre 1.4g, Calcium 93.6mg, Iron 1.1mg.

1. Preheat the oven to 180°C /350°F. Line an 80ml muffin tray with paper cases.

2. Combine the flour, baking powder, pumpkin (squash), spinach, fetta, paprika and rosemary in a large bowl and mix well.

3. In a smaller bowl, whisk the egg, butter and lactose-free milk. Gradually combine the flour mixture with the egg mixture without overmixing.

4. Divide the mixture among the paper cases. Once the mixture has been divided evenly, sprinkle the muffins with pepitas.

5. Bake for 20-25 minutes.
    To determine whether the muffins are cooked through, insert a skewer into the centre to see if it comes out clean.
    Remove from the oven and transfer the muffins to a wire rack to cool. Serve warm or at room temperature.

PANCAKES

SERVES 4

1 cup plain low FODMAP flour
3 tsp baking powder
¼ tsp salt
1½ tbsp castor sugar
1½ tbsp vegetable oil
1 egg
1 tsp vanilla extract
¾ cup lactose-free milk
butter or oil for greasing
maple syrup to serve

Energy 1125kJ/269 Calories, Protein
4.6g, Total Fat 10.8g, Saturated Fat 2.5g,
Carbohydrate 38.4g, Sugars 8.9g, Dietary
fibre 0.5g, Calcium 68.0mg, Iron 0.7mg.

1. Sift the flour, baking powder and salt into a mixing bowl.
   Add the sugar.

2. Make a well in the centre of the flour mixture. Add the oil, egg
   and vanilla essence. With a stirring spoon, gradually stir the
   flour into the liquid

3. Add the milk and mix into a smooth batter, adding extra milk if
   required. If possible, allow the batter to stand for 1-2 hours in
   the fridge.

4. Preheat a frypan over medium heat and grease the pan with
   butter. For each pancake, pour ¼ cup of batter into the frypan,
   spreading it into a round (you should be able to fit two to three
   in a frypan).

5. Cook the pancakes until bubbles appear on the surface. Flip
   the pancakes when the underside is golden. Remove them from
   the pan and repeat with the remaining batter.

6. Serve the pancakes hot with maple syrup.

SERVING SUGGESTION

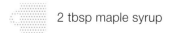 2 tbsp maple syrup

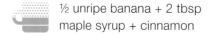 ½ unripe banana + 2 tbsp
maple syrup + cinnamon

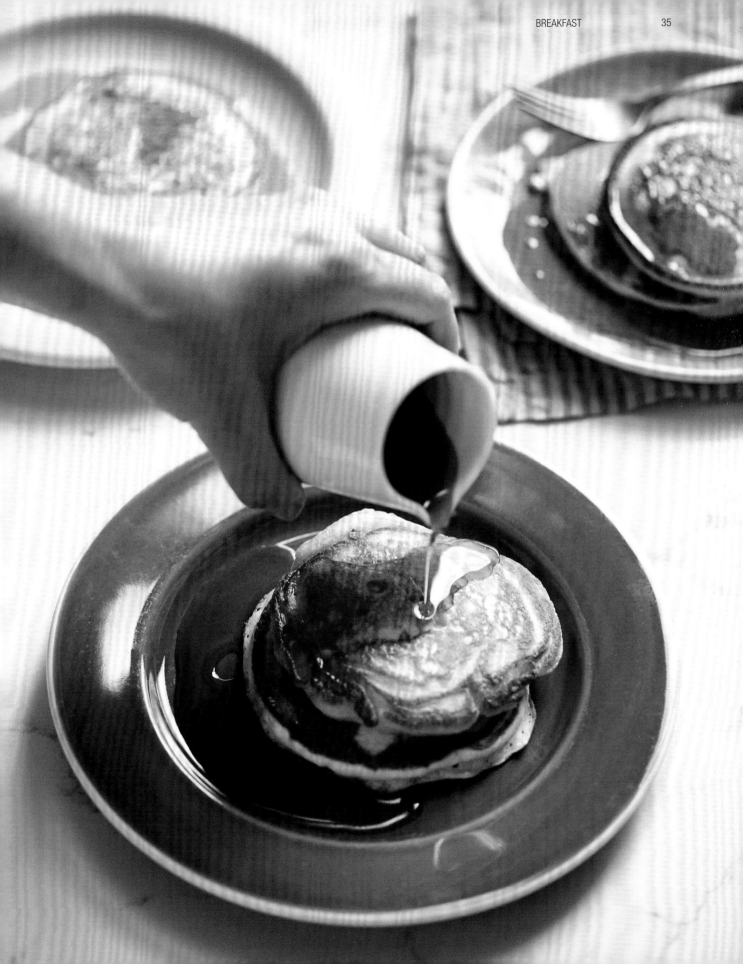

CINNAMON CHOC CHIP OVERNIGHT OATS

SERVES 1

½ cup rolled oats
¼ cup lactose-free yoghurt
½ cup lactose-free milk
1 tsp chia seeds
½ tsp cinnamon
¼ tsp cocoa powder
1 tsp vanilla essence (extract)
1 tbsp dark chocolate chips
½ firm banana, sliced

1. Add all ingredients (excluding banana) to a jar or bowl and stir to combine. Cover and refrigerate overnight.

2. To serve, top the oats with sliced banana.

Energy 1954 kJ/467 Calories, Protein 15.6g, Total Fat 18.6g, Saturated Fat 9.0g, Carbohydrate 55.3g, Sugars 23.5g, Dietary fibre 8.0g, Calcium 299.0mg, Iron 3.1mg.

STRAWBERRY AND WALNUT OVERNIGHT OATS

SERVES 1

½ cup rolled oats
½ cup lactose-free milk
¼ cup lactose-free yoghurt
1 tsp chia seeds
½ cup strawberries, sliced
1 tsp maple syrup
½ tsp vanilla essence
10g (½oz) walnuts, roughly chopped

1. Add all ingredients to a jar or bowl and stir to combine.

2. Cover the jar and refrigerate overnight.

3. Serve cold or at room temperature.

Energy 1554kJ/371 Calories, Protein 14.3g, Total Fat 13.5g, Saturated Fat 5.2g, Carbohydrate 44.6g, Sugars 18.5g, Dietary fibre 7.4 g, Calcium 294.8mg, Iron 2.4mg.

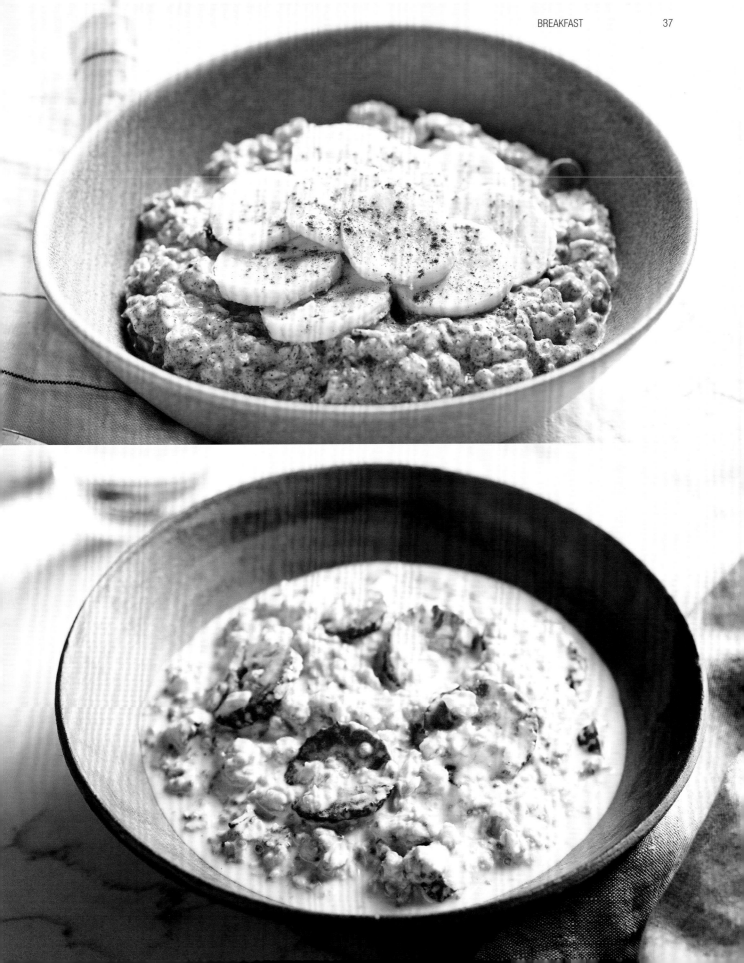

WALNUT, SEED AND COCONUT GRANOLA

SERVES 16

3 cups rolled oats

1¼ cups walnuts, roughly chopped

¼ cup linseeds

¼ cup pumpkin seeds or pepitas

¼ cup chia seeds

1 tsp ground cinnamon

½ cup coconut oil, melted

½ cup maple syrup

1 tsp vanilla essence (extract)

½ cup coconut flakes

¼ cup dried cranberries,
    roughly chopped

Energy 1011kJ/242 Calories, Protein
4.3g, Total Fat 19.4g, Saturated Fat 9.4g,
Carbohydrate 13.3g, Sugars 9.8g, Dietary
fibre 3.4g, Calcium 70.4mg, Iron 1.0mg.

1. Preheat the oven to 180°C/350°F. Line a baking tray with baking paper.

2. In a large mixing bowl, combine the oats, walnuts, linseeds, pumpkin seeds, chia seeds and cinnamon.

3. Add the melted coconut oil, maple syrup and vanilla essence. Mix well until coated.

4. Pour the granola onto the baking tray and press down evenly with the back of a spoon.

5. Bake for 10 minutes, then remove the granola from the oven, break it up with a spoon, and re-compress into an even layer. Bake for another 10 minutes or until light golden.

6. Remove from the oven and add the coconut flakes. Bake for a further 2-3 minutes or until lightly toasted.

7. Allow the granola to cool for at least 45 minutes then stir in the dried cranberries.

8. Store the granola in an airtight container at room temperature for up to 2 weeks.

SERVING SUGGESTION

 ½ cup lactose free
milk or yoghurt

 1 cup unsweetened
almond milk

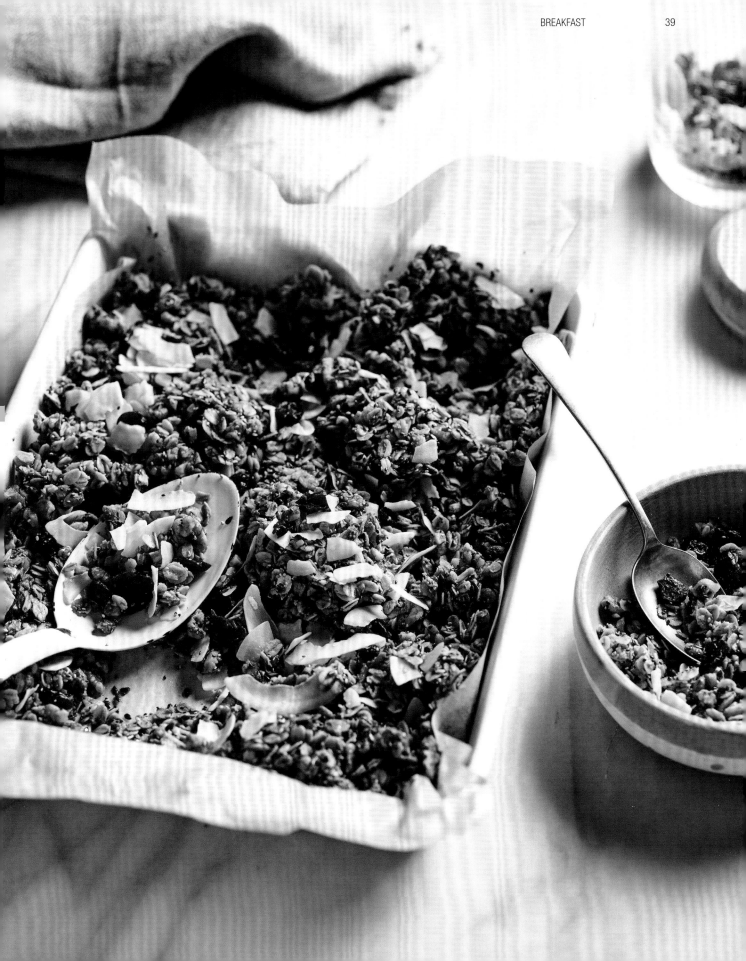

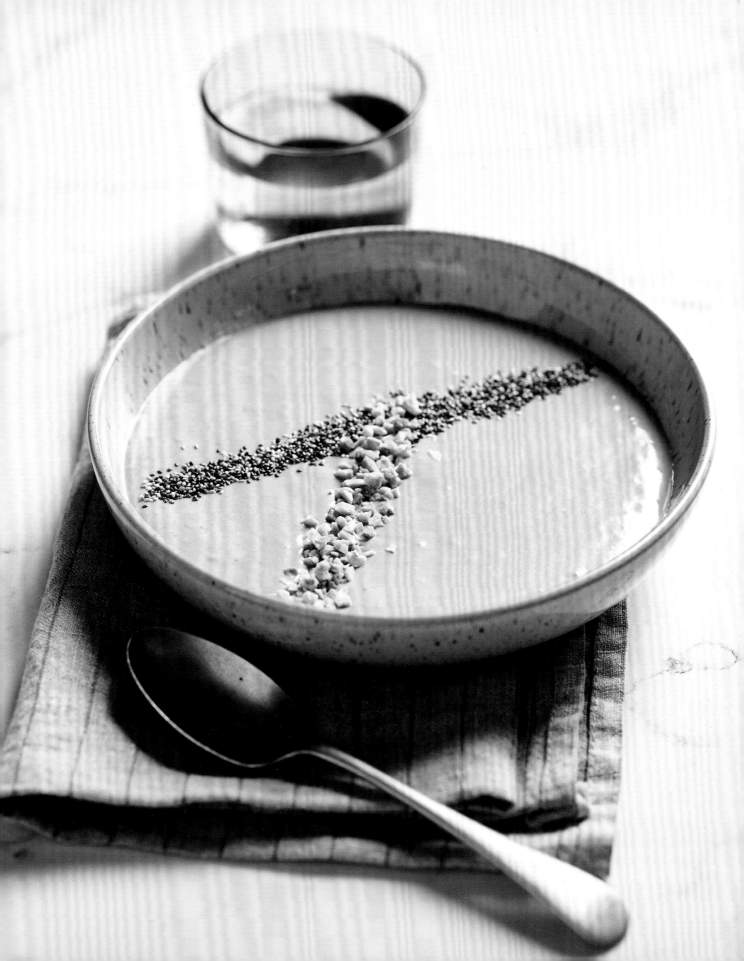

CACAO SMOOTHIE BOWL

SERVES 1

1 firm banana, peeled and frozen

⅓ cup almond milk (calcium-fortifed)

1 tbsp natural peanut butter

2 tbsp coconut yoghurt

2 tsp cacao powder

1 tsp chia seeds

1 cup ice

1 tsp chia seeds to garnish

1 tbsp crushed peanuts to garnish

Energy 2169kJ/518 Calories, Protein 14.1g,
Total Fat 35.6g, Saturated Fat 16.2g,
Carbohydrate 32.2g, Sugars 20.8g, Dietary
fibre 8.5g, Calcium 284.2mg, Iron 2.7mg.

1. Place all ingredients except garnishes into a blender or food processor and blitz until smooth.

2. Garnish with chia seeds and peanuts. Serve immediately.

GREEN SMOOTHIE

SERVES 1

1 cup baby spinach

1 cup frozen pineapple, chopped

½ cup lactose-free milk

¼ cup lactose-free yoghurt

1 tsp chia seeds

½ frozen firm banana

1. Add all ingredients to a blender and blitz until smooth. Serve immediately.

Energy 1176kJ/281 Calories, Protein 10.5g, Total Fat 7.6g, Saturated Fat 4.2g, Carbohydrate 38.0g, Sugars 33.5g, Dietary fibre 6.8g, Calcium 337.0mg, Iron 1.7mg.

BANANA BREAD SMOOTHIE

SERVES 1

1 small firm banana, peeled, sliced and frozen

½ cup unsweetened almond milk (calcium-fortified)

¼ cup rolled oats

¼ cup lactose-free yoghurt

½ tsp vanilla essence

½ tsp cinnamon

½ tsp nutmeg

1 tsp maple syrup

1. Add all ingredients to a blender and blitz until smooth and creamy. Serve immediately.

Energy 1203kJ/287 Calories, Protein 7.7g, Total Fat 7.7g, Saturated Fat 2.0g, Carbohydrate 43.9g, Sugars 25.8g, Dietary fibre 4.7g, Calcium 202.2mg, Iron 1.2mg.

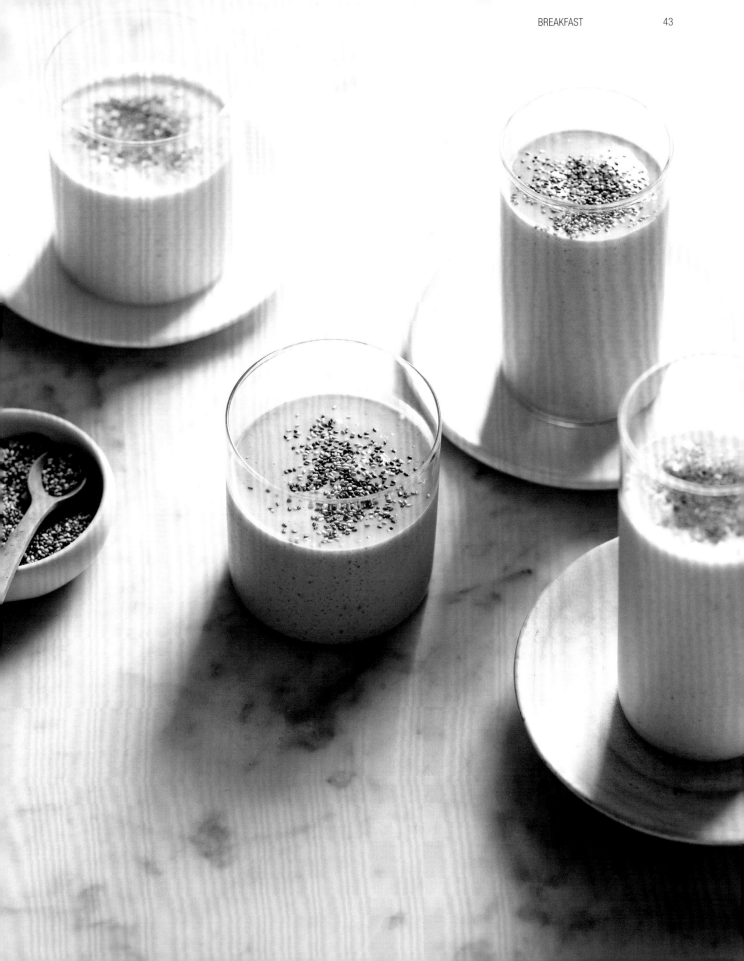

GREENS BREAKFAST PIE

SERVES 6

2 tbsp garlic-infused olive oil

130g (4½oz) leek greens, finely sliced

75g (2½oz) Tuscan kale, stems
    removed and coarsely chopped

1 cup parsley, roughly chopped

6 eggs

¼ cup lactose-free cream

1 tsp Dijon mustard

1 lemon, zested

salt to taste

pepper to taste

60g (2oz) butter, melted

6 sheets filo pastry

30g (1oz) parmesan

Energy 1253kJ/299 Calories, Protein
11.3g, Total Fat 23.7g, Saturated Fat 8.8g,
Carbohydrate 10.0g, Sugars 1.8g, Dietary
fibre 1.9g, Calcium 122.3mg, Iron 1.7mg.

1. Preheat the oven to 180°C/350°F.

2. In a large frypan over medium heat, heat the garlic-infused oil. Add the leeks and cook for approximately 4 minutes or until softened, stirring occasionally. Add the kale and cook, stirring often, for approximately 2 minutes or until wilted. Add the parsley and stir to combine. Set aside to cool.

3. In a medium-sized bowl, whisk together the eggs, cream, mustard, lemon zest, salt and pepper until combined. Set aside.

4. Oil a 24–26cm (9–10 inch) pie dish or shallow casserole. Place the filo on a clean surface and use a dry tea towel to cover the pastry. Layer a damp tea towel over the dry towel to prevent the filo from drying out.

5. Brush a sheet of filo with melted butter and place it in the pie dish with the edges hanging over the sides. Brush another sheet of filo with butter and place it at right angles to the first sheeet. Continue until all the filo and butter are used, brushing the final layer of filo with butter.

6. Arrange the greens mixture over the filo. Pour in the egg mixture and sprinkle over the grated parmesan. Fold the edges of the filo towards the centre to partly cover the filling. Bake for 40 minutes or until the filo is golden.

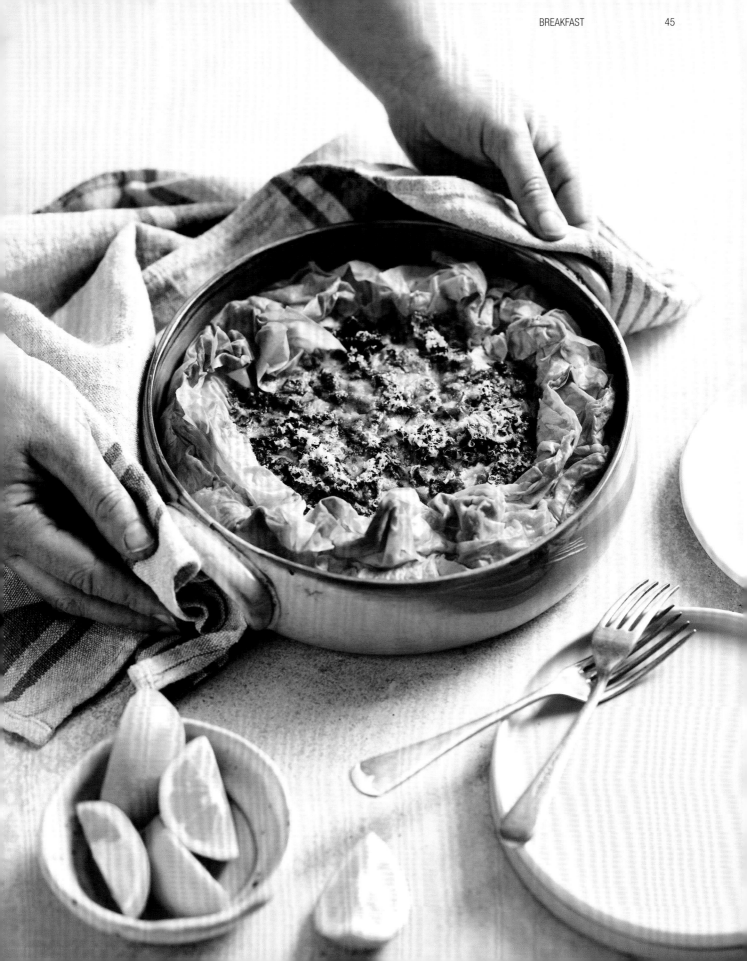

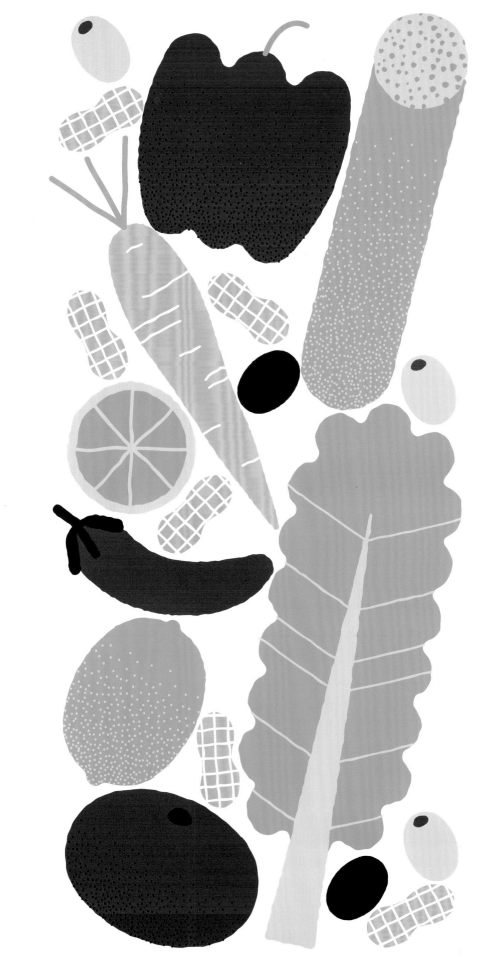

SALADS

FATTOUSH SALAD

SERVES 4

DRESSING
1½ tsp sumac
¼ tsp salt
¼ tsp black pepper
¼ cup lemon juice
½ tbsp balsamic vinegar
1½ tbsp olive oil
1 tsp garlic-infused olive oil

SPICED CORN TORTILLA TRIANGLES
3–4 corn tortillas
olive oil spray
½ tsp sumac
½ tsp smoked paprika

SALAD
200g (7oz) cos lettuce leaves, trimmed
   and chopped
2 medium-sized tomatoes, core
   removed and diced
1 medium-sized Lebanese cucumber,
   halved lengthwise and cut into 1cm
   (½ inch) slices
½ cup spring onions (scallions) (green
   tops only)
3 radishes, finely sliced
half a medium-sized green capsicum
   (bell pepper), deseeded and cut into
   2cm (¾ inch) cubes
½ cup mint leaves, roughly chopped
½ cup parsley leaves, roughly chopped

Energy 869kJ/208 Calories, Protein 4.0g,
Total Fat 11.5g, Saturated Fat 1.7g,
Carbohydrate 19.0g, Sugars 6.3g, Dietary
fibre 5.5g, Calcium 89.5mg, Iron 2.3mg.

1. Preheat the oven to 200°C/400°F. Line an oven tray with
    baking paper.

2. To make the dressing, combine the sumac, salt, black pepper,
    lemon juice, balsamic vinegar and both olive oils in a jar and
    shake. Ensure all of the ingredients are well combined.

3. To make the toasted tortillas, cut each tortilla into eight triangles
    and spread onto the oven tray. Spray lightly with olive oil and
    sprinkle with sumac and smoked paprika. Bake for 8–10
    minutes or until crisp and golden. Set aside.

4. To make the salad, place all of the vegetables and herbs into a
    large bowl. Add the dressing and toss well with your hands.

5. Add the tortillas immediately before serving.

SERVING SUGGESTION

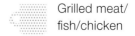 Grilled meat/
fish/chicken

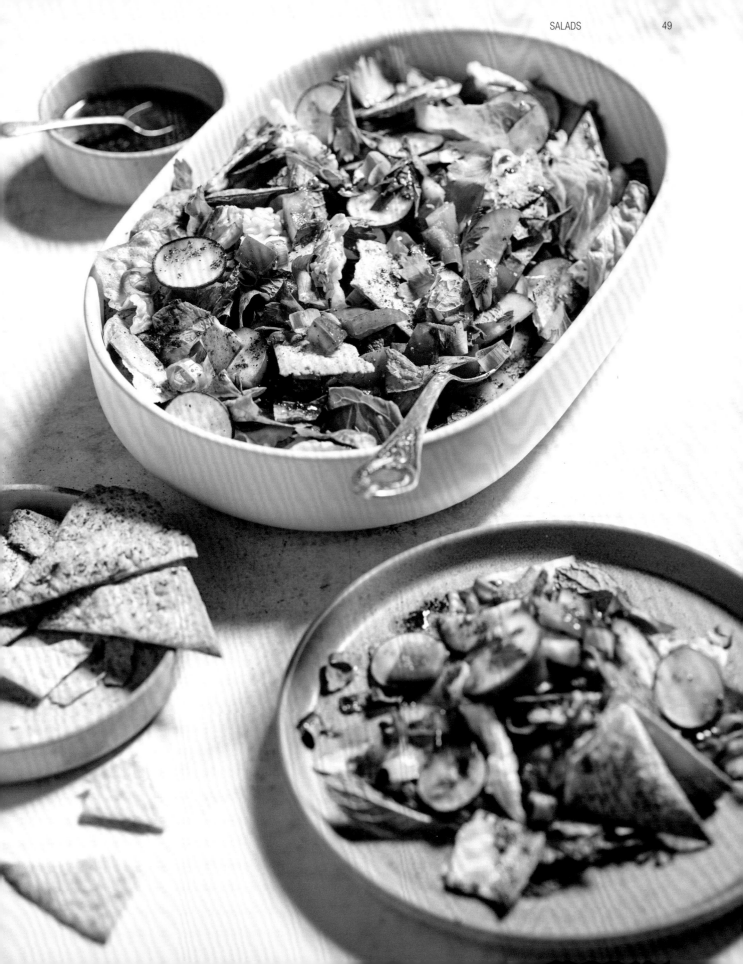

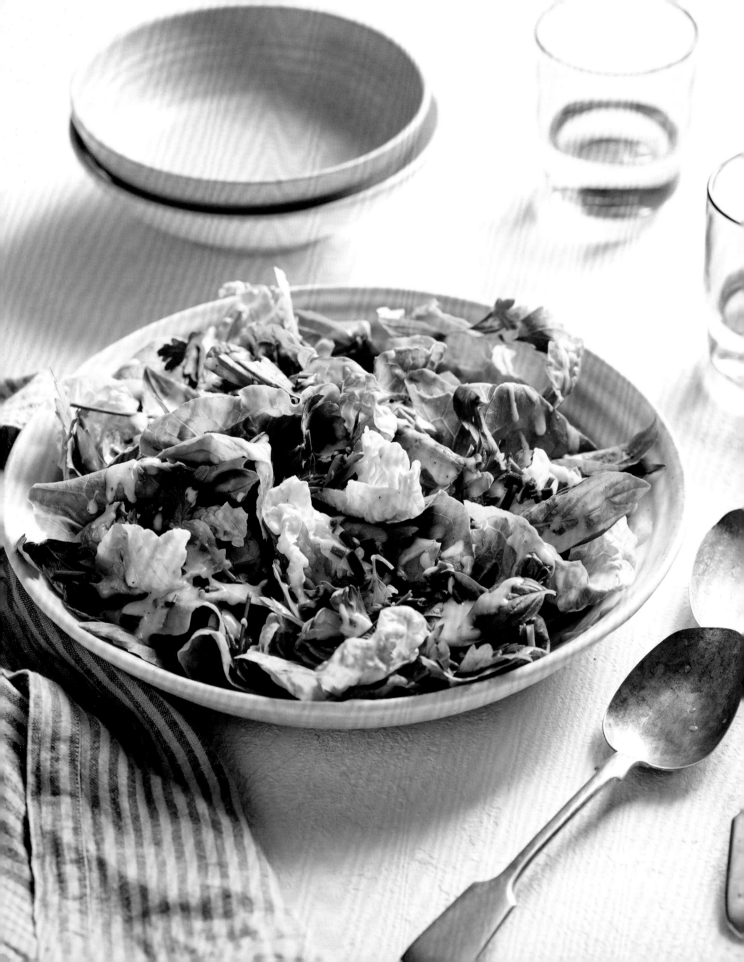

FRENCH GREEN SALAD

SERVES 4

1 butter lettuce head

half a cos lettuce head

1 tbsp parsley

1 tbsp basil

1 tbsp fresh chives

French dressing to serve
   (see 'basics', page 228)

Energy 340kJ/81 Calories, Protein 1.3g,
Total Fat 7.7g, Saturated Fat 1.2g,
Carbohydrate 1.2g, Sugars 1.1g, Dietary
fibre 1.5g, Calcium 30.8mg, Iron 0.8mg.

1. Separate the lettuce leaves (butter and cos) and wash and dry in salad spinner. Tear the larger leaves in half.

2. Remove the fresh parsley and basil leaves from stems. Tear the basil leaves and chop the chives.

3. Place the French dressing in the bottom of a large salad serving bowl. Add the lettuce and herbs.

4. Just before serving, use your hands to gently toss the lettuce and herbs until the leaves are well covered with dressing. Serve immediately.

SERVING SUGGESTION

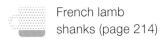 French lamb shanks (page 214)

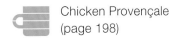 Chicken Provençale (page 198)

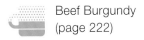 Beef Burgundy (page 222)

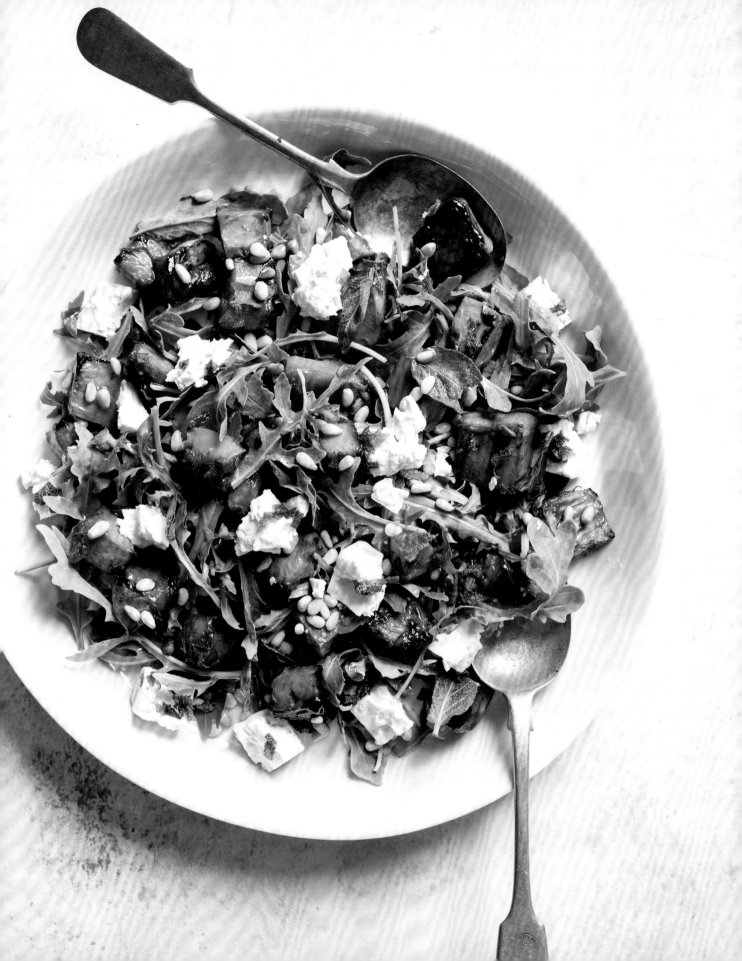

ROASTED PUMPKIN AND FETTA SALAD

SERVES 4

¼ cup olive oil

2 tbsp maple syrup

1 tbsp sage, finely chopped

1 kent pumpkin (squash), peeled and
cut into 2cm (¾ inch) cubes (3 cups)

2 cups rocket leaves (arugula)

2 tbsp pine nuts, toasted

100g (3½oz) fetta, crumbled

Energy 1332kJ/318 Calories, Protein
7.2g, Total Fat 25.5g, Saturated Fat 6.6g,
Carbohydrate 14.6g, Sugars 13.2g, Dietary
fibre 3.8g, Calcium 215.1 mg, Iron 1.7mg.

1. Preheat the oven to 220°C/425°F.

2. Combine the oil, maple syrup and sage in a bowl. Add the
    pumpkin to the bowl and toss to coat.

3. Spread the pumpkin (squash) out evenly onto a tray lined with
    baking paper and bake for 25 minutes or until golden brown.
    Set aside to cool.

4. In a salad bowl, toss the pumpkin with the rocket (arugula)
    and pine nuts. Top with crumbled fetta to serve.

SERVING SUGGESTION

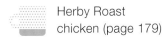 Herby Roast
chicken (page 179)

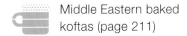 Middle Eastern baked
koftas (page 211)

GREEN PAPAYA SALAD

SERVES 6

⅓ cup lime juice

2 tbsp brown sugar

1 tbsp fish sauce

15 green beans

1 medium-sized green
 papaya (pawpaw)

10 cherry tomatoes, halved

½ cup coriander (cilantro),
 roughly chopped

1 fresh red chilli, finely sliced

2 tbsp peanuts, roughly chopped

Energy 338kJ/81 Calories, Protein 2.2g,
Total Fat 1.9g, Saturated Fat 0.3g,
Carbohydrate 11.6g, Sugars 11.3g, Dietary
fibre 3.9g, Calcium 48.8mg, Iron 1.2mg.

1. To make the dressing, combine the lime juice, brown sugar
    and fish sauce in a small bowl and set aside.

2. Cook the green beans in a small saucepan of boiling water for
    approximately 5 minutes. Rinse with cold water and cut into
    2cm (¾ inch) pieces.

3. Peel and grate the papaya (pawpaw), discarding the seeds
    and membrane, and place the flesh in a large salad bowl.

4. Add the tomatoes, coriander (cilantro), chilli and beans.

5. Pour the dressing over the salad and toss to combine.
    Sprinkle with peanuts to serve.

SERVING SUGGESTION

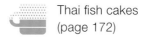 Thai fish cakes
(page 172)

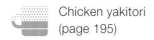 Chicken yakitori
(page 195)

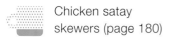 Chicken satay
skewers (page 180)

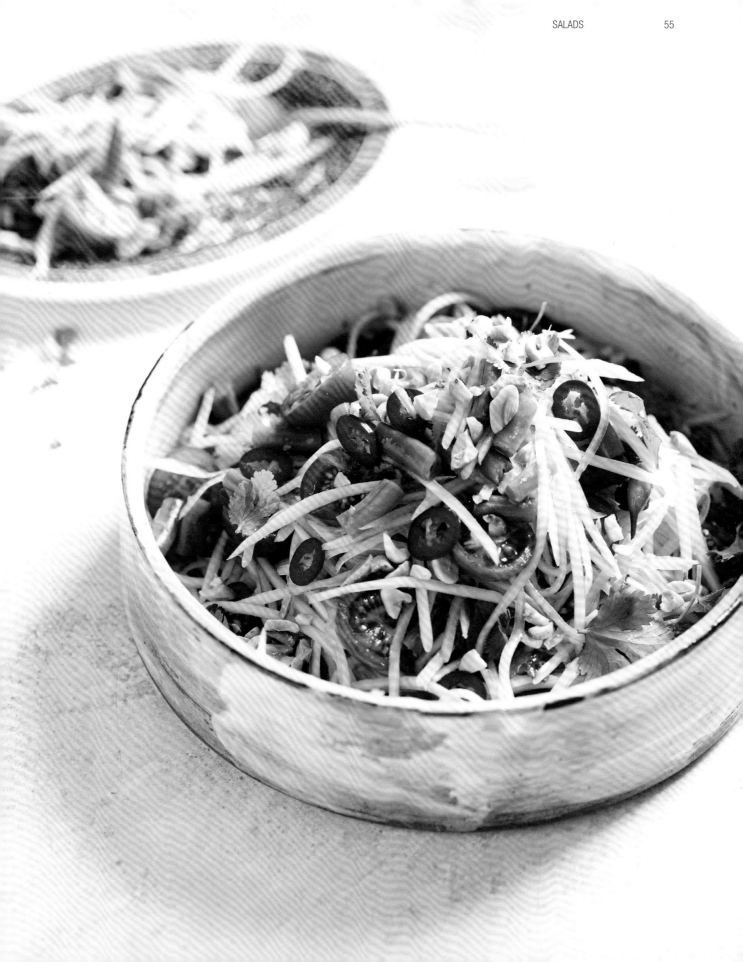

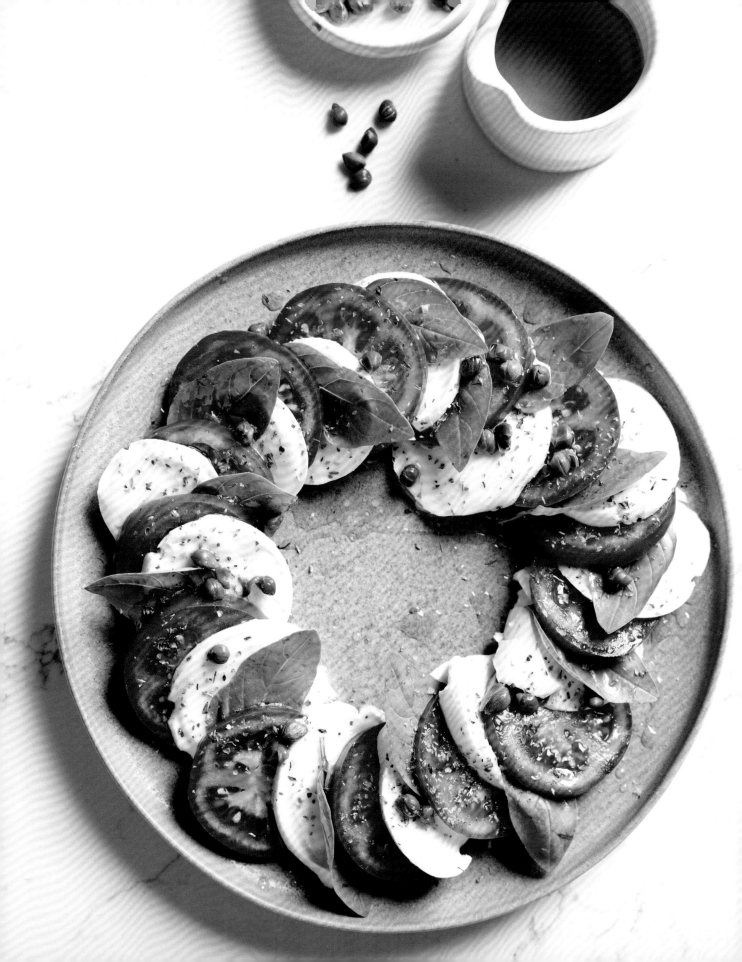

CAPRESE SALAD

SERVES 6

6 medium-sized fresh tomatoes
(common/truss), sliced
2 large buffalo mozzarella balls
(125g/4½oz each), thickly sliced
¼ cup basil leaves
2 tbsp white wine vinegar
2 tbsp olive oil
sea salt to taste
ground black pepper to taste
1 tbsp baby capers
½ tsp dried oregano

Energy 867kJ/207 Calories, Protein 7.9g,
Total Fat 16.9g, Saturated Fat 7.6g,
Carbohydrate 4.9g, Sugars 4.0g, Dietary
fibre 1.9g, Calcium 312.5mg, Iron 0.5mg.

1. Arrange the tomato, mozzarella and basil attractively on a flat serving dish.

2. Dress the salad with vinegar and olive oil. Garnish with salt, pepper, capers and oregano to serve.

SERVING SUGGESTION

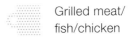 Grilled meat/
fish/chicken

JAPANESE POTATO SALAD

SERVES 4

half a medium-sized cucumber

1 carrot

salt to taste

500g (1lb) potatoes

5 eggs

6 cornichons

2 slices of ham

85g (3oz) Japanese mayonnaise

½ tsp mustard

½ bunch chives, finely chopped

Energy 1453kJ/347 Calories, Protein 14.4g, Total Fat 22.9g, Saturated Fat 4.4 g, Carbohydrate 19.8g, Sugars 2.9g, Dietary fibre 2.7g, Calcium 53.5mg, Iron 2.3mg.

1. Peel the potatoes and cut into 3cm (1¼ inch) pieces. Add the potatoes to a saucepan and cover with water. Bring to a simmer and cook for 25–30 minutes or until the potatoes are tender.

2. Meanwhile, cut the cucumber and carrot in half lengthways and slice thinly into half-moons. Sprinkle with salt and set aside for approximately 20 minutes to soften.

3. Rinse the cucumber and carrot under cold water to remove the salt. Set aside.

4. Remove the potatoes with a slotted spoon and set aside to cool. Keep the water in the saucepan.

5. Bring the water to a boil and add the eggs. Cook the eggs for 10 minutes then transfer them to a bowl of cold water to cool. Peel the eggs, cut into quarters and set aside.

6. Slice the cornichons and thinly slice the ham into strips.

7. Combine the mayonnaise and mustard in a large salad bowl. Using a fork, mix in the cooked potatoes, roughly breaking up the potatoes to give the salad a fluffy texture.

8. Add the cucumbers, carrots, cornichons, ham and eggs to the bowl and mix. Adjust the seasoning to taste.

9. Serve sprinkled with chives.

SERVING SUGGESTION

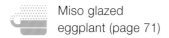
Miso glazed eggplant (page 71)

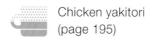
Chicken yakitori (page 195)

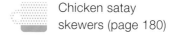
Chicken satay skewers (page 180)

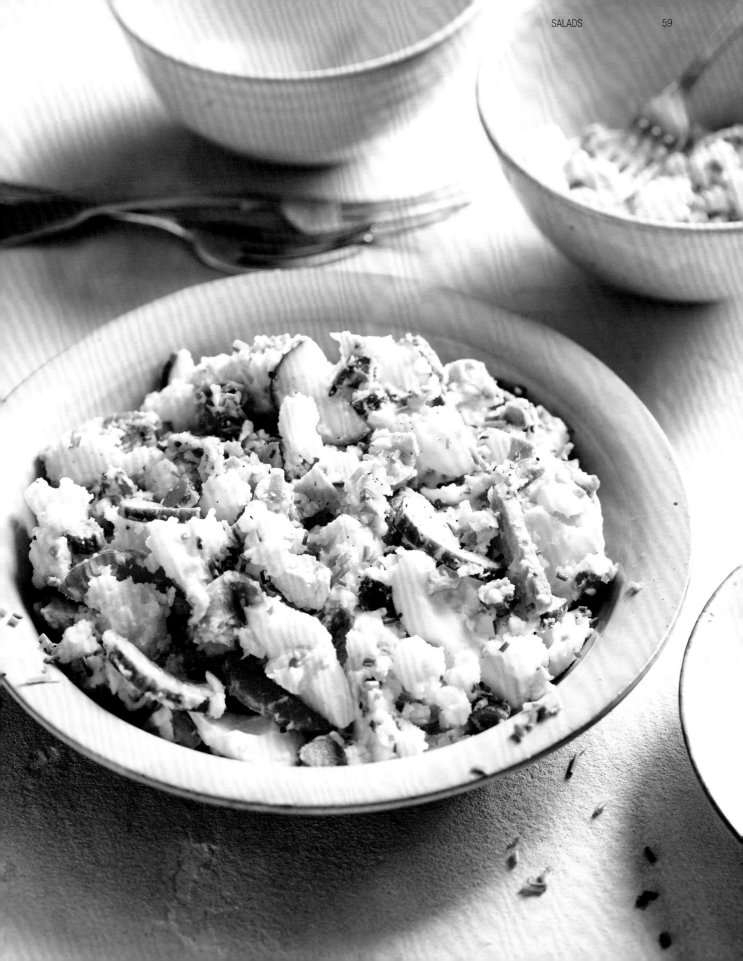

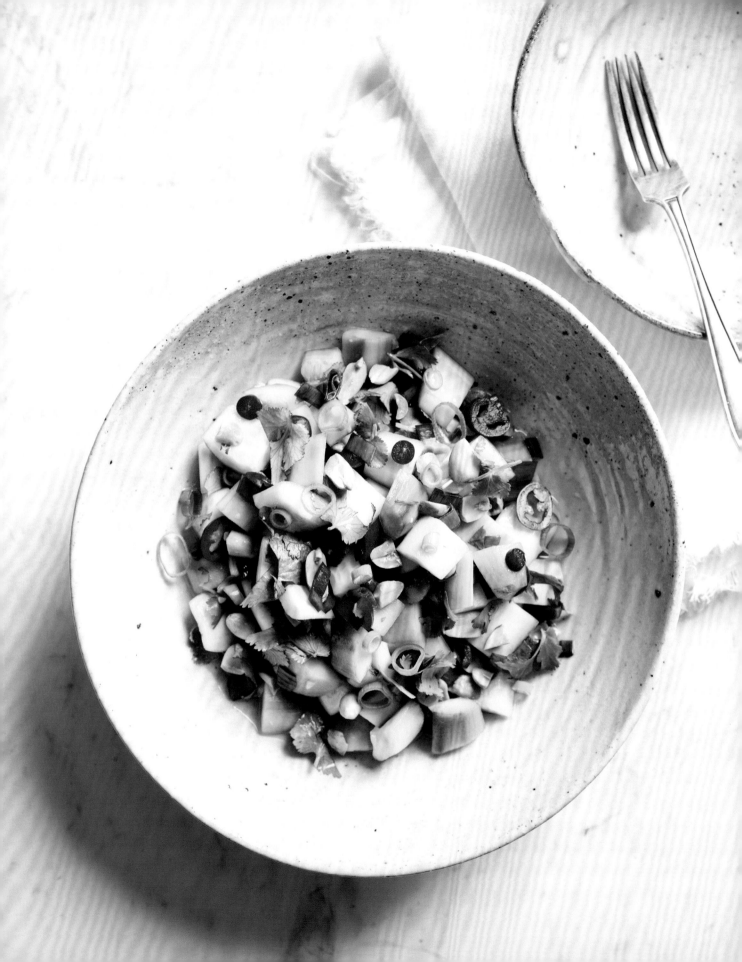

SPICY THAI CUCUMBER SALAD

SERVES 5

2 medium-sized cucumbers

1 tbsp caster sugar

2 tbsp white vinegar

1 fresh red chilli or to taste, finely
chopped

50g (2oz) roasted peanuts, chopped

½ cup spring onions (scallions) (green
tops only), finely chopped

¼ cup fresh coriander (cilantro),
chopped

¼ tsp fish sauce

Energy 374 kJ/89 Calories, Protein 3.6g,
Total Fat 4.9g, Saturated Fat 0.8g,
Carbohydrate 6.2g, Sugars 5.8g, Dietary
fibre 3.0g, Calcium 29.3mg, Iron 0.8mg.

1. Peel the cucumbers, cut in half lengthways and remove the
   seeds. Slice into 1cm (½ inch) pieces.

2. Combine the sugar and vinegar in a bowl until the sugar
   dissolves. Add the cucumber and mix well.

3. Add the finely chopped red chillies, peanuts, spring onion tops
   (scallions) and coriander leaves (cilantro) to the bowl. Mix well.

4. Place the bowl in the refrigerator for 30–60 minutes. Stir in the
   fish sauce just before serving.

SERVING SUGGESTION

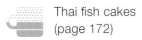
Thai fish cakes
(page 172)

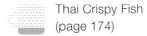
Thai Crispy Fish
(page 174)

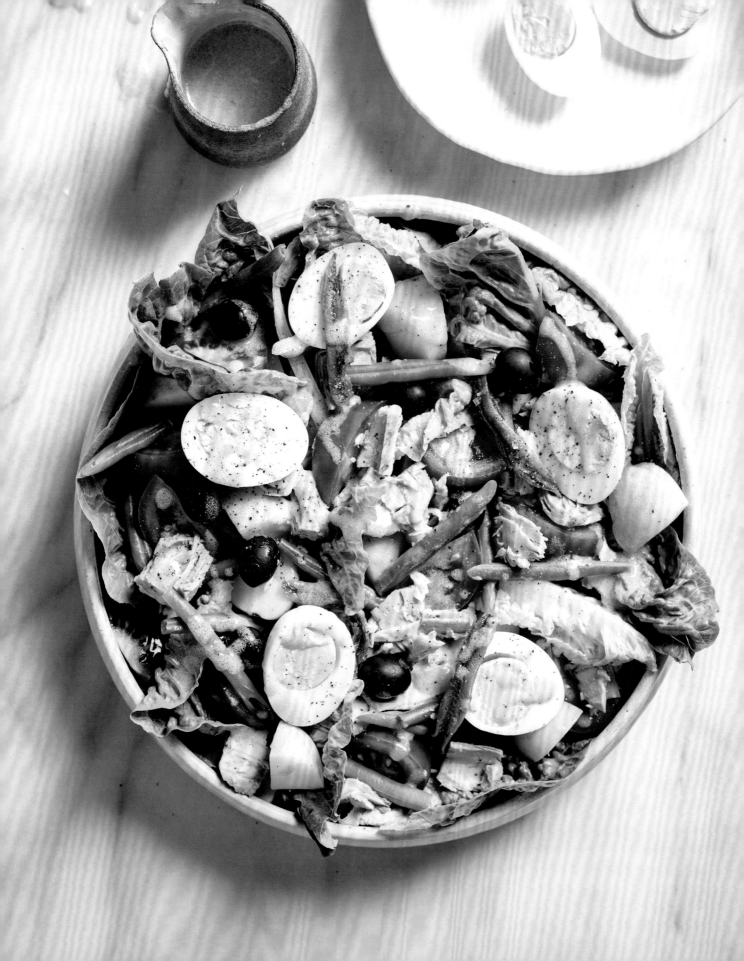

SALAD NICOISE

SERVES 4

12 small potatoes, boiled

4 eggs, hard boiled

150g (5oz) green beans, trimmed

300g (10½oz) cos lettuce

2 tomatoes (common/truss), sliced
    into wedges

¾ cup black olives

425g (15oz) canned tuna chunks

3 anchovy fillets

French dressing to serve (see 'basics',
    page 228)

Energy 1584kJ/379 Calories, Protein
40.8g, Total Fat 11.8 g, Saturated Fat 2.9g,
Carbohydrate 23.5g, Sugars 5.8g, Dietary
fibre 5.4g, Calcium 88.7mg, Iron 4.3mg.

1. To blanch the beans, add them to a large pot of boiling water and cook for 2–3 minutes or until the beans turn bright green in colour but are still crisp. Drain quickly and tip the beans into a bowl of iced water. Set aside for 4–5 minutes, then drain again.

2. Assemble the cos lettuce leaves, potatoes, blanched green beans, tomatoes, olives, tuna and anchovy fillets in a salad bowl. Pour over the French dressing just before serving.

TABOULI

SERVES 4

1 cup quinoa

⅓ cup lemon juice

3 tbsp extra virgin olive oil

3 cups parsley, finely chopped

1 ½ cups mint, finely chopped

1 ½ cups spring onions (scallions)
(green tops only), roughly chopped

1 medium-sized Lebanese
cucumber, sliced

1 medium-sized tomato (common/
truss), diced

Energy 1334kJ/318 Calories, Protein
6.8g, Total Fat 16.8g, Saturated Fat 2.5g,
Carbohydrate 31.0g, Sugars 4.6g, Dietary
fibre 7.4g, Calcium 92.2mg, Iron 2.6mg.

1. Cook the quinoa according to packet instructions and set aside
    to cool.

2. Combine the lemon juice and olive oil and set aside.

3. Combine the quinoa, herbs, spring onion (scallion) tops,
    cucumber and tomato in a large serving bowl.

4. Add the dressing just before serving and toss to combine.

SERVING SUGGESTION

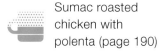 Sumac roasted
chicken with
polenta (page 190)

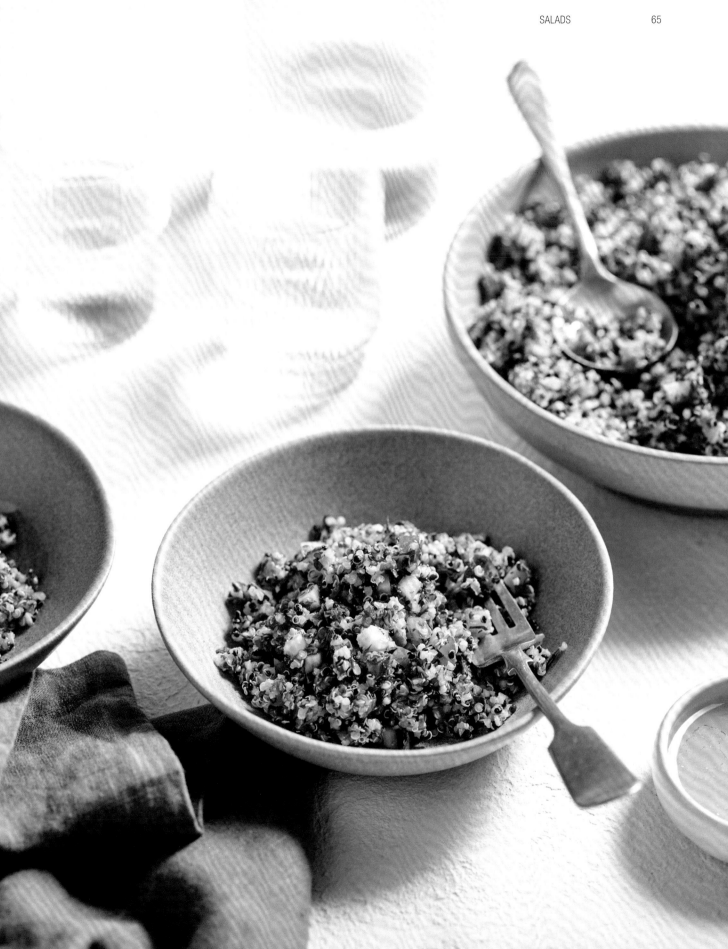

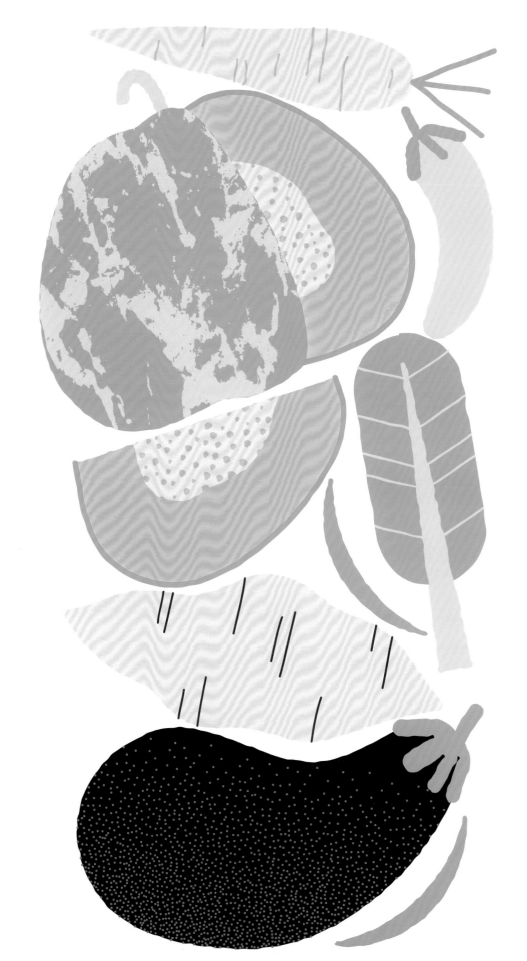

VEGETABLE SIDES

ROASTED VEGETABLES WITH BALSAMIC

SERVES 4

half a medium-sized red capsicum
   (bell pepper)
half a medium-sized green capsicum
   (bell pepper)
1 medium-sized potato
150g (5oz) zucchini (courgette)
⅓ medium-sized sweet potato
2 tbsp garlic-infused olive oil
2 tbsp balsamic vinegar
1 tsp rosemary leaves
½ tsp salt, or to taste

Energy 687kJ/164 Calories, Protein 3.1g,
Total Fat 9.5g, Saturated Fat 1.4 g,
Carbohydrate 14.8g, Sugars 7.1g, Dietary
fibre 3.2g, Calcium 22.8mg, Iron 0.8 mg.

1. Cut the red and green capsicum (bell pepper), potato, zucchini (courgette) and sweet potato into large pieces (approximately 2cm (¾ inch) in diameter).

2. Preheat the oven to 200°C/400°F.

3. In a bowl, combine the garlic-infused olive oil, balsamic vinegar, rosemary leaves and salt. Add the vegetables and mix well with your hands to ensure all the vegetables are well coated with the seasoning.

4. Spread all the vegetables except the zucchini on a large oven tray, leaving the excess seasoning behind. Cook for approximately 40–60 minutes or until the vegetables are tender and slightly charred. Add the zucchini for the final 15 minutes of cooking time.

5. Cool the vegetables slightly before serving.

SERVING SUGGESTION

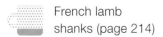
French lamb
shanks (page 214)

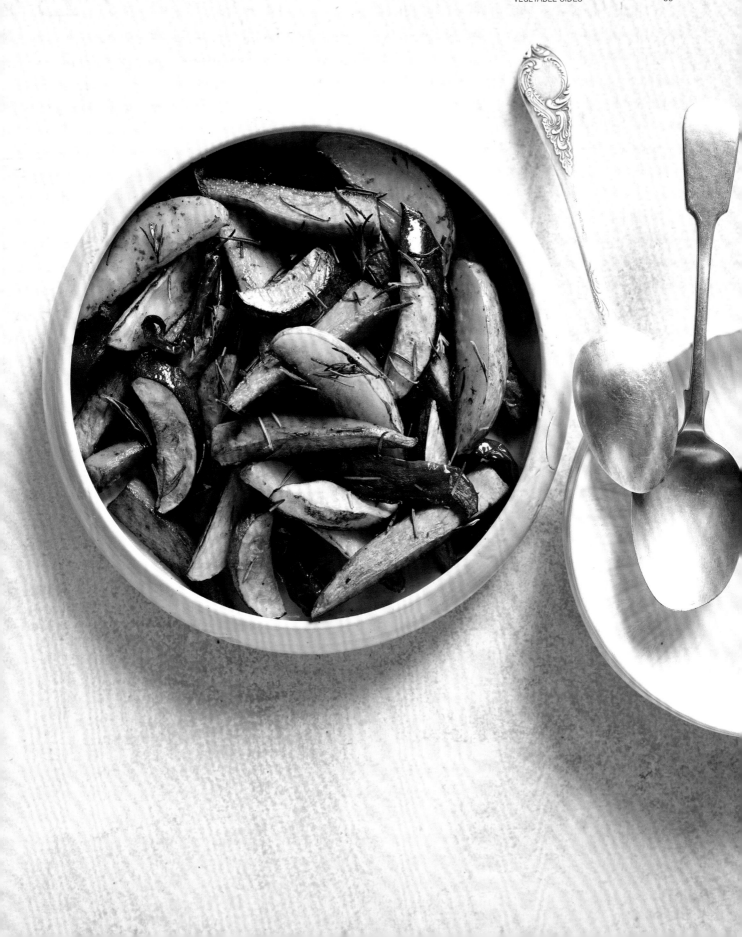

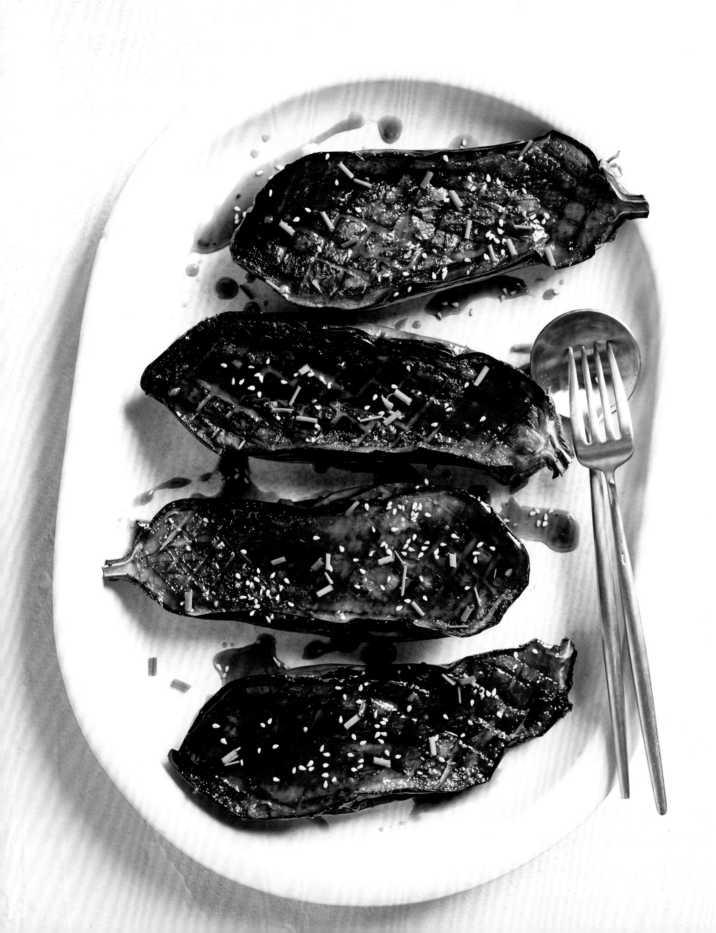

MISO GLAZED EGGPLANT

SERVES 4

2 medium-sized eggplants (aubergine)
   (700g/1lb 5oz)
vegetable oil for shallow frying
2 tbsp miso paste
1 tbsp mirin
1 tbsp white sugar
1 tsp rice wine vinegar
½ tbsp water
1 tbsp toasted sesame seeds
1 tsp chives, finely chopped

Energy 1606kJ/384 Calories, Protein
5.0g, Total Fat 32.1g, Saturated Fat 4.1g,
Carbohydrate 15.7g, Sugars 14.2g, Dietary
fibre 7.1g, Calcium 70.2mg, Iron 0.9mg.

1. Cut the eggplants (aubergine) in half lengthways. Score the flesh approximately 5mm deep in a criss-cross pattern.

2. Add oil to a depth of approximately 1cm (½ inch) to a deep-sided frying pan and heat over medium heat until the oil shimmers.

3. Add the eggplants to the pan, cut side down, and fry for approximately 5 minutes or until tender. Carefully remove the eggplant from the oil and drain well on a paper towel.

4. Whisk together the miso paste, mirin, sugar, rice wine vinegar and water in a small bowl until the sugar dissolves.

5. Preheat a griller or oven grill to 200°C/400°F. Spread the miso sauce onto the scored side of each eggplant. Place under the grill for approximately 5-10 minutes or until the glaze bubbles and begins to brown.

6. Serve sprinkled with sesame seeds and chives.

SERVING SUGGESTION

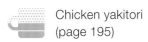
Chicken yakitori
(page 195)

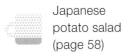
Japanese
potato salad
(page 58)

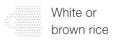
White or
brown rice

CHINESE BROCCOLI WITH OYSTER SAUCE

SERVES 4

600g (1lb 3oz) Chinese broccoli,
   trimmed
2 tbsp oyster sauce
1 tsp garlic-infused olive oil
1 tsp sesame oil
1 tbsp soy sauce
1 tsp olive oil
½ tsp salt

Energy 298kJ/71 Calories, Protein 2.1g,
Total Fat 4.5g, Saturated Fat 0.7g,
Carbohydrate 3.8g, Sugars 3.1 g, Dietary
fibre 3.3g, Calcium 137.2mg, Iron 1.3 mg.

1. Combine the oyster sauce, garlic-infused olive oil, sesame oil and soy sauce in a small bowl. Set aside.

2. Add the olive oil and salt to a saucepan of water and bring to the boil. Add the Chinese broccoli and cook for 2 minutes or until cooked to your liking.

3. Drain the Chinese broccoli, return it to the saucepan and add the sauce mixture. Toss to combine and serve immediately.

SERVING SUGGESTION

Baked fish with ginger, sesame and soy (page 168)

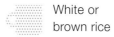
White or brown rice

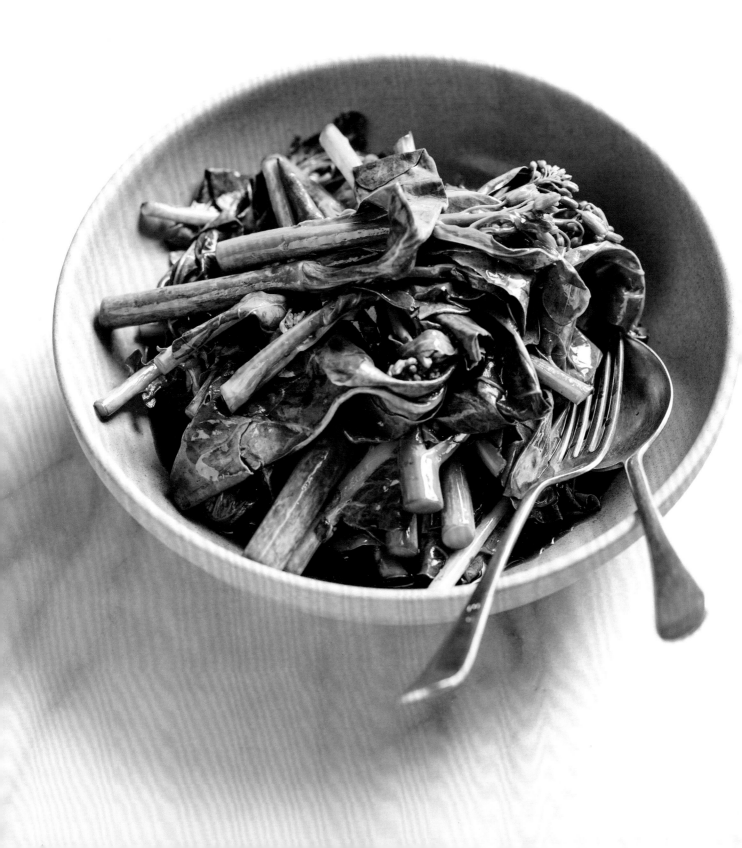

SLOW-ROASTED TRUSS TOMATOES

SERVES 4

2 tsp toasted caraway seeds

1 tsp salt

4 medium-sized tomatoes
   (common/truss)

3 tbsp extra virgin olive oil

sea salt flakes to taste

ground black pepper to taste

1 tsp dried oregano

Energy 640kJ/153 Calories, Protein 1.2g,
Total Fat 14g, Saturated Fat 2.2g,
Carbohydrate 4.7g, Sugars 3.8g, Dietary
fibre 2.4g, Calcium 35.4mg, Iron 0.8mg.

1. Preheat the oven to 130°C/270°F.

2. Finely grind the caraway seeds and salt in a mortar and
    pestle to make the caraway salt. Set aside.

3. Place the tomatoes on a tray with a wire rack. Drizzle the
    tomatoes with 2 tbsp of olive oil. Sprinkle with salt, pepper
    and oregano.

4. Bake for 2 hours.

5. Remove from the oven and assemble the tomatoes on a platter.
    Drizzle with the remaining 1 tbsp of olive oil, and season with
    caraway salt and additional pepper.

SERVING SUGGESTION

Herby roast chicken
(page 179)

Crispy roasted
rosemary potatoes
(page 83)

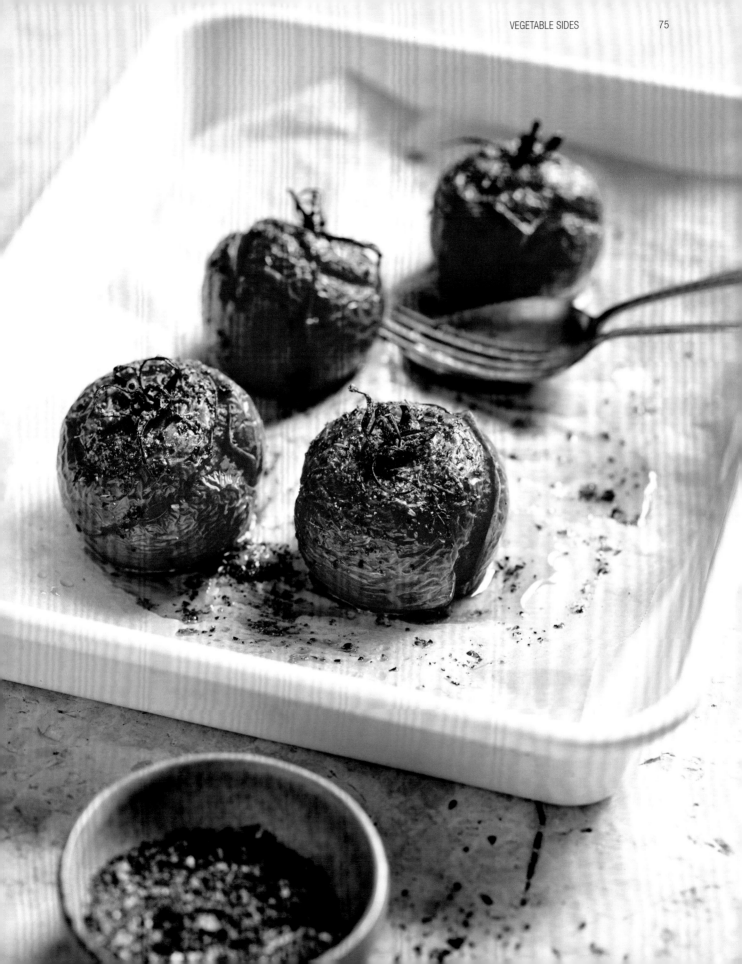

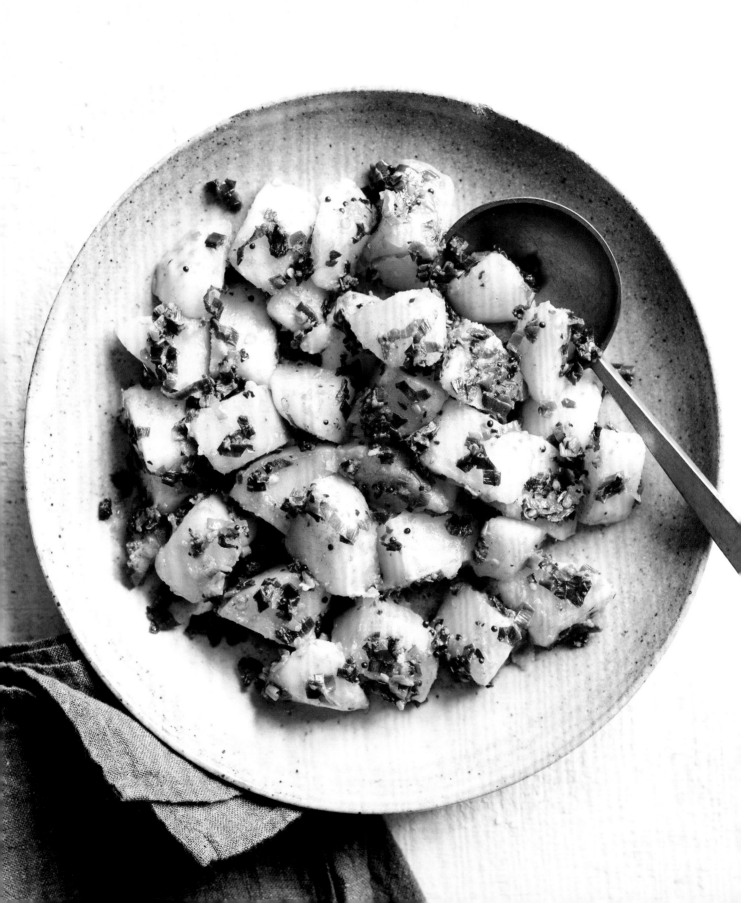

INDIAN POTATO CURRY

SERVES 4

500g (1lb) potatoes, peeled and halved

1 cup spring onions (scallions)
(green tops only), finely chopped

2 tbsp garlic-infused olive oil

¼ tsp black mustard seeds

½ tsp turmeric powder

½ tsp dried chillies, crushed

salt to taste

Energy 730kJ/174 Calories, Protein 3.5g,
Total Fat 9.5g, Saturated Fat 1.4g,
Carbohydrate 17.4g, Sugars 0g, Dietary
fibre 2.1g, Calcium 14.0mg, Iron 1.2mg.

1. Cook the potatoes in boiling water until just cooked. Drain and set aside to cool.

2. Heat the garlic-infused olive oil in a heavy-based saucepan. Add the spring onion tops and black mustard seeds.

3. Cook over low heat until soft, stirring occasionally and taking care not to burn.

4. Add the turmeric, chilli and salt. Stir well.

5. Add the potatoes and cook until heated through, stirring to coat them with the spices. Serve hot.

SERVING SUGGESTION

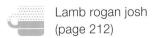 Lamb rogan josh
(page 212)

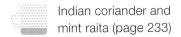 Indian coriander and
mint raita (page 233)

CHINESE STYLE EGGPLANT

SERVES 4

1 medium-sized eggplant (aubergine), cut into strips
½ tsp salt
1 tbsp garlic-infused olive oil
1 tsp light soy sauce
1 tsp dark soy sauce
½ tsp sugar
1 tsp black vinegar
3 tbsp water
½ tsp cornflour (cornstarch)
2 tbsp vegetable oil
1 medium-sized green capsicum (bell pepper), deseeded and cut into strips
1 tbsp ginger, finely chopped
1 large red chilli, finely sliced
2 tbsp spring onions (scallions) (green tops only), finely chopped
2 tbsp coriander (cilantro)

Energy 687kJ/164 Calories, Protein 2.4g, Total Fat 14.2g, Saturated Fat 1.7g, Carbohydrate 5.3g, Sugars 4.9g, Dietary fibre 4.0g, Calcium 33.9mg, Iron 0.7mg.

1. Season the eggplant (aubergine) with salt and set aside for 20 minutes.

2. To make the sauce, combine the garlic-infused olive oil, light and dark soy sauce, sugar, black vinegar, water and cornflour (cornstarch) in a bowl.

3. Heat 1 tbsp of the vegetable oil in a wok over medium-high heat. Add the eggplant and stir-fry until soft. Add the capsicum (bell pepper) and cook for 1 minute. Remove the vegetables from the wok and set aside.

4. Add half the vegetable oil and the ginger and chilli to the wok and stir-fry until fragrant.

5. Add the soy sauce mixture and stir-fry for 1 minute or until the sauce thickens.

6. Add the eggplant and capsicum and stir-fry for approximately 1-2 minutes or until the sauce thickens further.

7. Serve garnished with spring onion tops (scallions) and coriander (cilantro).

SERVING SUGGESTION

 Kung pao chicken (page 189)

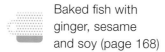 Baked fish with ginger, sesame and soy (page 168)

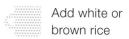 Add white or brown rice

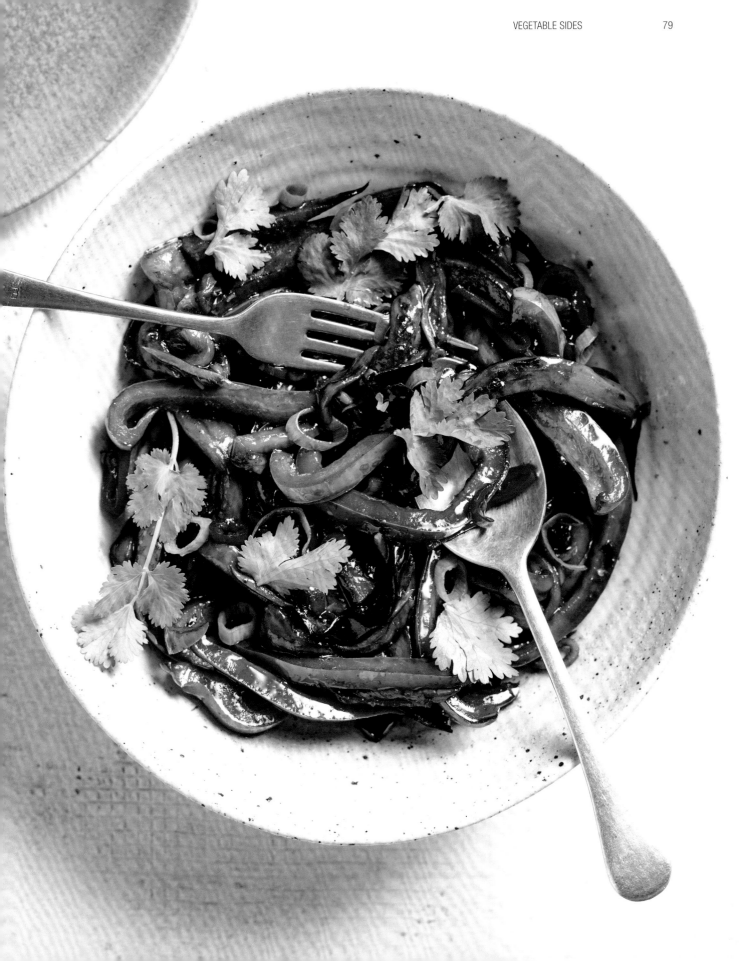

ROASTED GREEN AND RED CAPSICUM

SERVES 4

2 medium-sized green capsicums
   (bell peppers)
1 medium-sized red capsicum
   (bell pepper)
olive oil spray
4 tbsp garlic-infused olive oil
6 mint leaves, chopped
salt flakes to taste
2 tbsp flat-leaved parsley,
   roughly chopped
flat-leaved parsley and mint leaves
   to serve
20g (1oz) pecorino cheese
   (or parmesan), shaved into ribbons

Energy 1046kJ/250 Calories, Protein
6.0g, Total Fat 20.2g, Saturated Fat 3.7g,
Carbohydrate 8.9g, Sugars 8.7g, Dietary
fibre 5.7g, Calcium 68.9mg, Iron 1.4mg.

1. Preheat the griller or the oven grill function to 180°C/350°F. Line a baking tray with foil and spray with oil.

2. Place the capsicums (bell peppers) on the tray and grill for approximately 30 minutes on each side or until blackened.

3. Use tongs to remove the capsicums from the tray and place them in a plastic bag. Leave to cool for 1 hour.

4. Remove the blackened capsicum skins, which should lift off easily.

5. Halve the capsicums lengthways and scrape out seeds. Slice the capsicums into 2cm (¾ inch) strips and place in a mixing bowl.

6. Add the garlic-infused olive oil, mint, salt flakes and parsley. Gently toss to coat and set aside at room temperature for 2-3 hours before serving.

7. Arrange the capsicums on a serving dish and sprinkle with mint and parsley leaves and pecorino. Serve with fresh sourdough spelt bread (or another low FODMAP loaf).

SERVING SUGGESTION

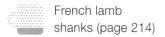
French lamb
shanks (page 214)

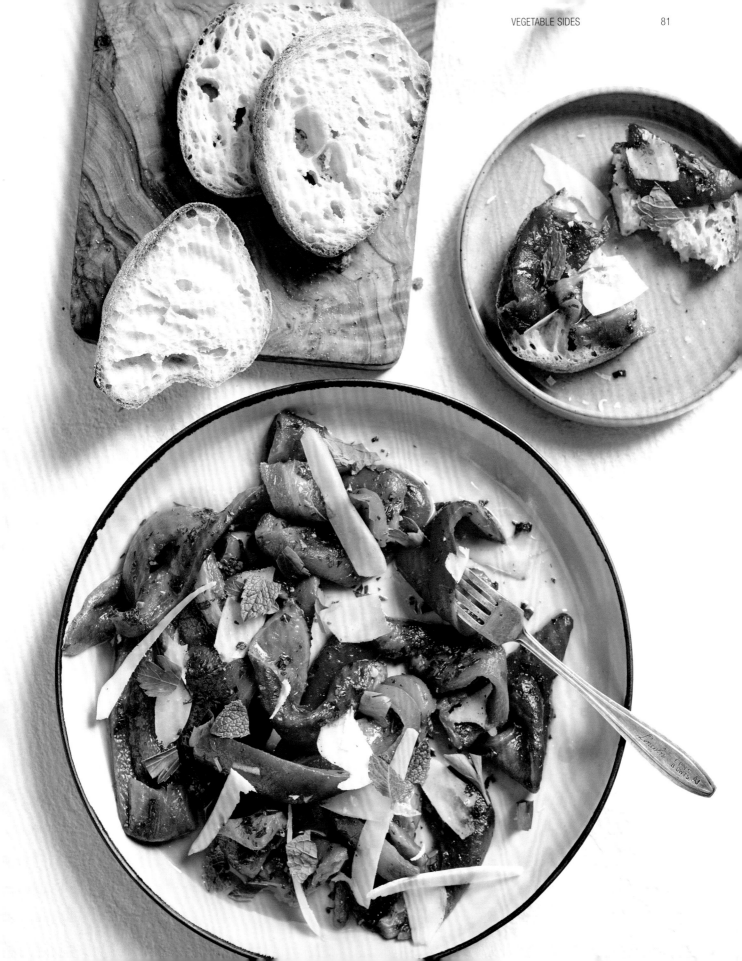

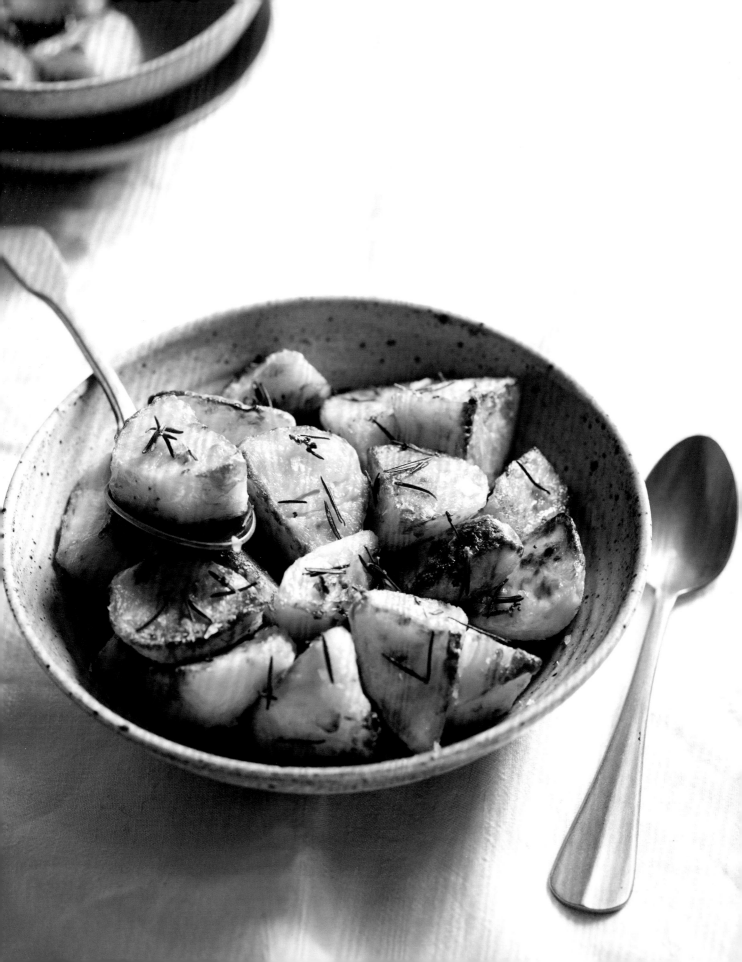

CRISPY ROASTED ROSEMARY POTATOES

SERVES 6
1kg (2lb 2oz) potatoes, peeled
2 tbsp olive oil
2 tbsp rosemary leaves
salt flakes to taste

Energy 995kJ/238 Calories, Protein 6.3g,
Total Fat 6.7g, Saturated Fat 1.0g,
Carbohydrate 34.8g, Sugars 1.0g, Dietary
fibre 5.7g, Calcium 10.0mg, Iron 1.4mg.

1. Preheat the oven to 200°C/390°F.

2. Cut the potatoes into quarters and cook in a large pot of simmering water and cook for 15 minutes or until the potatoes are tender. Drain well.

3. Return the potatoes to the pot. Lightly shake the potatoes in the pot to roughen up the edges. This will mean crisp outsides once roasted.

4. Place the oil into a heavy-based roasting dish and heat in the oven for 5 minutes.

5. Add the potatoes and toss to coat them in the oil.

6. Scatter the rosemary leaves over the potatoes and bake for 30 minutes. Turn the potatoes over and roast for an additional 30 minutes or until golden brown.

7. Remove from the oven and season with salt while hot. Serve immediately.

SERVING SUGGESTION

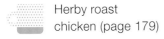 Herby roast chicken (page 179)

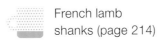 French lamb shanks (page 214)

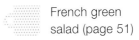 French green salad (page 51)

THAI VEGETABLE STIR-FRY

SERVES 5

½ cup coconut milk

2 tbsp fish sauce

1 tbsp lime juice

½ tsp chilli flakes

2 tsp brown sugar

1 tbsp garlic-infused olive oil

¼ cup spring onions (scallions)
(green tops only), finely chopped

2½cm (1 inch) piece galangal,
finely sliced

1 red chilli, sliced

1 carrot, sliced

300g (10½oz) broccoli, heads only

1 medium-sized green capsicum
(bell pepper), sliced

15 green beans

150g (5oz) bok choy,
roughly chopped

2 tbsp Thai basil leaves

Energy 522kJ/125 Calories, Protein 5.1g,
Total Fat 8.0g, Saturated Fat 3.8g,
Carbohydrate 6.0g, Sugars 5.7 g, Dietary
fibre 4.8g, Calcium 40.9mg, Iron 1.2mg.

1. To make the stir-fry sauce, combine the coconut milk, fish sauce, lime juice, chilli flakes and brown sugar in a bowl. Stir until the sugar dissolves.

2. Heat the oil in a wok or frypan over medium-high heat.

3. Add the spring onion tops (scallion), galangal and chilli and stir-fry for 1-2 minutes.

4. Add the carrot, broccoli, and sauce to the pan and fry for 3-4 minutes.

5. Add the capsicum (bell pepper) and green beans and let simmer for 1 minute.

6. Lastly, add the bok choy and simmer until cooked.

7. Remove the pan from heat. Scatter with Thai basil and serve with jasmine rice.

SERVING SUGGESTION

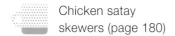 Chicken satay
skewers (page 180)

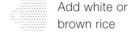 Add white or
brown rice

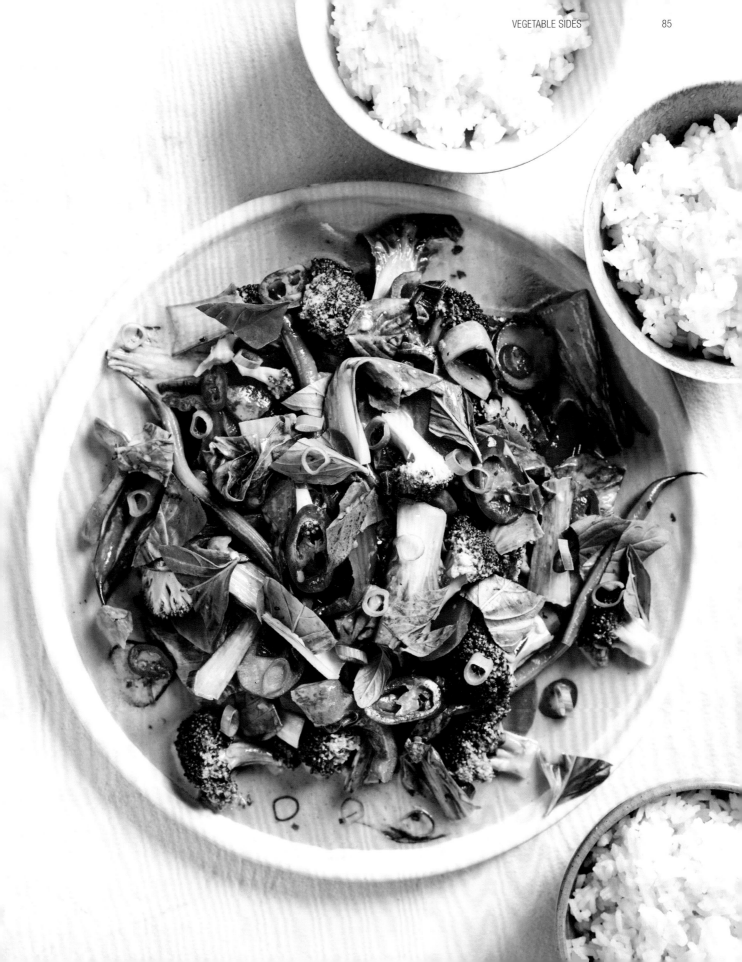

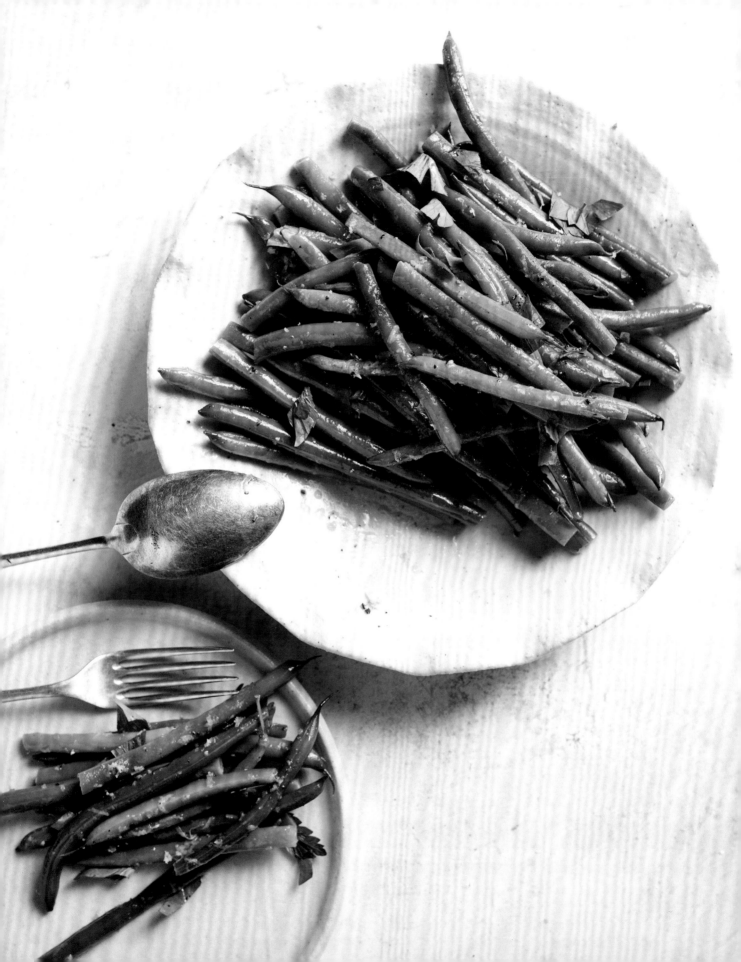

LEMON PARSLEY GREEN BEANS

SERVES 4
450g (1lb) green beans
1 tbsp butter
1 tbsp garlic-infused olive oil
1 tsp lemon zest
¼ cup parsley, chopped
salt and pepper to taste

Energy 278kJ/66 Calories, Protein 1.4g,
Total Fat 5.3g, Saturated Fat 1.4g,
Carbohydrate 2.5g, Sugars 2.0g, Dietary
fibre 2.2g, Calcium 39.2mg, Iron 0.6mg.

1. Bring a large pot of water to the boil.

2. Add the green beans and cook for 2-3 minutes or until the beans turn bright green in colour but are still crisp.

3. Drain quickly and tip the beans into a bowl of iced water. Set aside for 4–5 minutes, then drain again.

4. Preheat a heavy-based pan over medium heat and add the butter and oil. When the butter has melted, add the blanched green beans, lemon zest and chopped parsley and heat through for 1-2 minutes.

5. Season with salt and freshly ground pepper and serve.

SERVING SUGGESTION

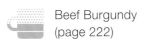 Beef Burgundy (page 222)

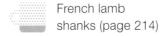 French lamb shanks (page 214)

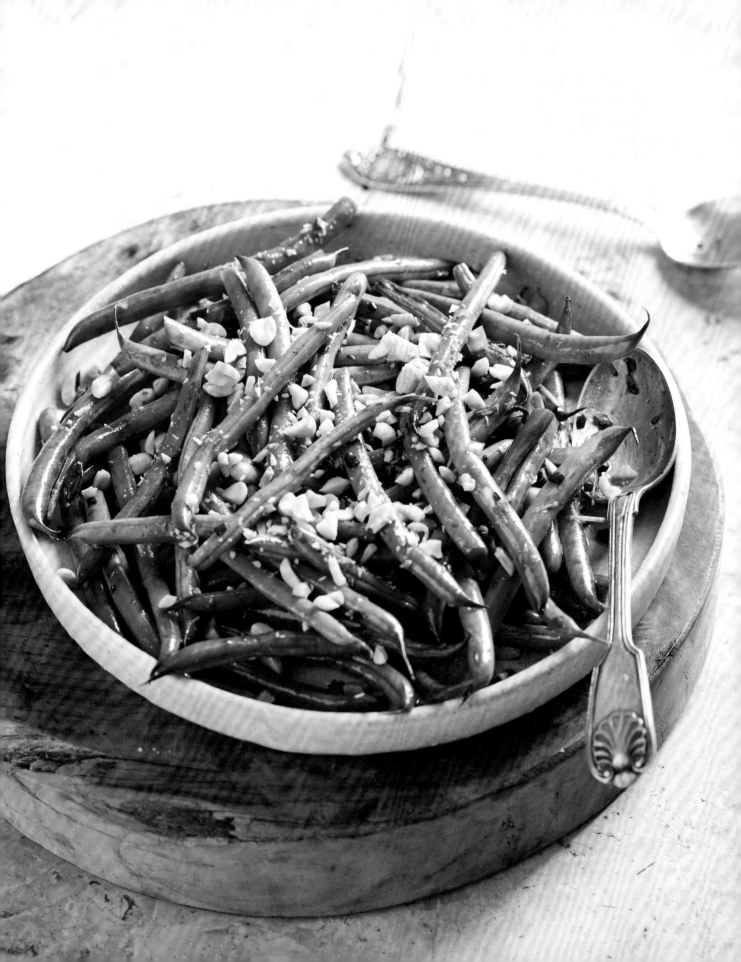

THAI GREEN BEANS

SERVES 5

1 red chilli, finely chopped
1 tbsp soy sauce
1 tbsp lime juice
½ tbsp brown sugar
1 tbsp rice wine vinegar
¼ cup water
1 tbsp garlic-infused olive oil
1 lemongrass stalk, finely chopped
500g (1lb) green beans
2 tbsp peanuts, roughly chopped

Energy 388kJ/93 Calories, Protein 3.2g,
Total Fat 5.8g, Saturated Fat 0.9g,
Carbohydrate 5.2g, Sugars 4.3g, Dietary
fibre 3.7g, Calcium 51.4mg, Iron 0.9mg.

1. Combine the chilli, soy sauce, lime juice, brown sugar and rice wine vinegar in a small bowl with the water. Set aside.

2. Heat the oil in a frypan over medium heat. Add the lemongrass and sauté for 2 minutes.

3. Add the green beans to the pan and sauté for 2 minutes.

4. Turn the heat to low and add the sauce mixture. Cover and simmer for 3 minutes, or until the green beans are tender.

5. Remove the lid and stir for an additional minute. Most of the liquid should have evaporated and the beans should be glazed with sauce.

6. Sprinkle with peanuts and serve.

SERVING SUGGESTION

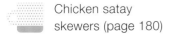 Chicken satay
skewers (page 180)

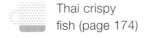 Thai crispy
fish (page 174)

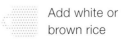 Add white or
brown rice

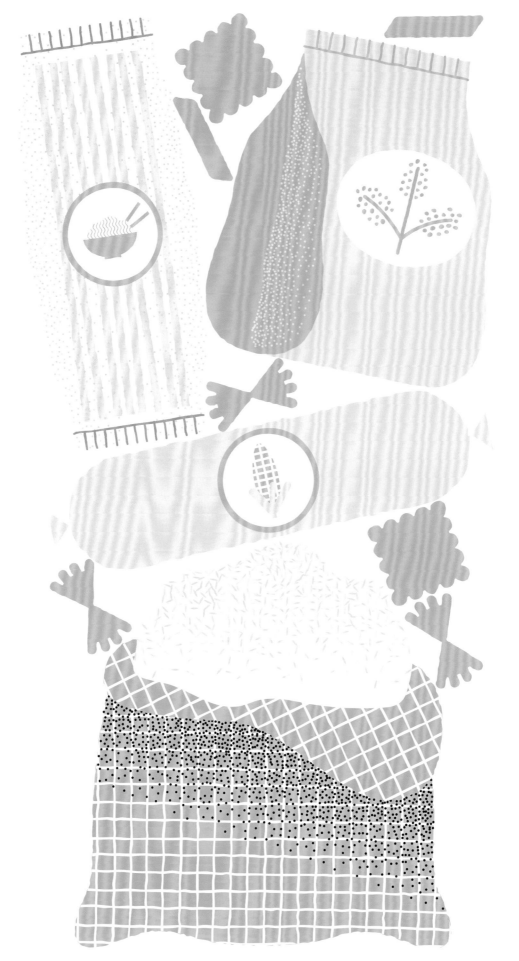

GRAINS

PAELLA

SERVES 4

1 tbsp garlic-infused olive oil

¼ cup spring onions (green tops only)

½ cup parsley

1 tsp sweet paprika

1 cup tinned tomato

salt to taste

¼ tsp pepper

2½ cups low FODMAP chicken stock

1 pinch saffron threads

1 tbsp extra-virgin olive oil

450g (1lb) boneless chicken thigh,
    roughly chopped into
    bite-sized pieces

300g (10½oz) arborio rice

450g (1lb) raw king prawns (shrimp),
    peeled and deveined (leave the
    tail intact)

120g (4oz) green beans, trimmed and
    cut in half

2 tbsp parsley

half a lemon, cut into wedges

Energy 2616kJ/625 Calories, Protein
49.7g, Total Fat 20.3g, Saturated Fat 4.7g,
Carbohydrate 58.6g, Sugars 2.2g, Dietary
fibre 2.3g, Calcium 191.3mg, Iron 2.5mg.

1. Combine the garlic-infused olive oil, spring onion tops (scallions), parsley, paprika, tomatoes, salt and pepper in a food processor. Process until a chunky tomato sauce forms. Set aside.

2. Place the chicken stock and saffron in a medium saucepan and bring to the boil, then simmer over medium-high heat for 5 minutes or until the saffron has infused and coloured the stock.

3. In a paella pan or large non-stick frypan, heat the extra-virgin olive oil over high heat. Add the chicken and cook for 3-5 minutes or until brown. Add the rice and cook, stirring, for 1 minute.

4. Add the stock and tomato sauce and bring to the boil.

5. Reduce the heat to low, add the prawns and cook for 15 minutes without stirring. If you are using a frypan, rotate the pan to ensure the rice cooks evenly. Increase heat to medium, add the green beans and cook for a further 4 minutes.

6. Remove the paella from the heat, cover the pan with foil and set aside for 5 minutes while the rice absorbs the liquid. Garnish with parsley and lemon wedges and serve.

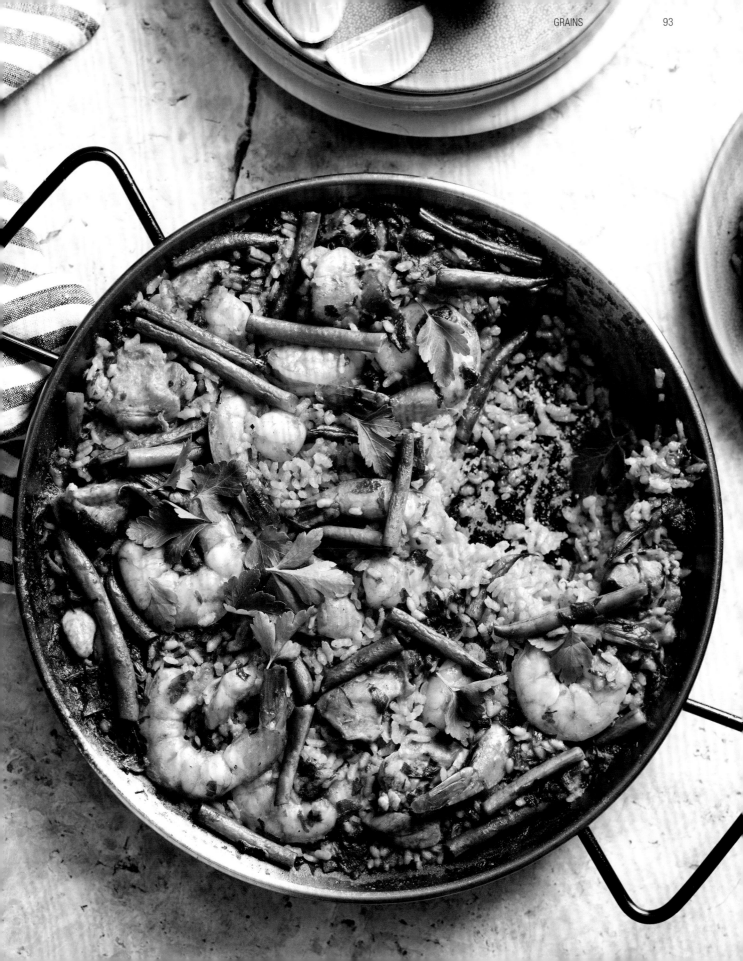

MUSHROOM RISOTTO

SERVES 4

500g (1lb) oyster mushrooms
1 low FODMAP chicken stock cube
5 cups water
2 tbsp garlic-infused olive oil
1 cup leek (green tops only),
    finely chopped
2 tbsp white wine vinegar
1½ cups arborio rice
½ cup dry white wine
60g (2oz) butter
½ cup finely grated parmesan
parsley leaves, to garnish
1 tbsp sour cream

Energy 2365kJ/565 Calories, Protein 15.0g,
Total Fat 27.8g, Saturated Fat 13.0g,
Carbohydrate 60.5g, Sugars 2.6g, Dietary
fibre 4.1g, Calcium 122.7mg, Iron 2.2mg.

1. Blitz half of the mushrooms in a food processor until coarsely chopped.

2. Add the stock cube and 5 cups of water to a saucepan and bring to the boil. Remove from the heat, cover to keep warm and set aside.

3. Heat the oil over medium heat in a separate pan, then add the leek tops. Sauté for 4 minutes then add the coarsely chopped mushroom. Cook for a further 4 minutes then add 1 tbsp of the vinegar.

4. Add the rice and wine and stir for 2-3 minutes. Gradually add the hot stock, stirring well after each addition, and allowing the rice to absorb the liquid before adding more. Once all the stock is added, the rice should be al dente.

5. Remove from the heat and add half the butter and half the parmesan. Set aside.

6. Roughly chop the remaining mushrooms.
Melt the remaining butter in a frypan over medium-high heat, add the mushrooms and cook for 4 minutes or until golden. Stir in the remaining vinegar.

7. Serve the risotto topped with mushrooms, sour cream, parsley and parmesan.

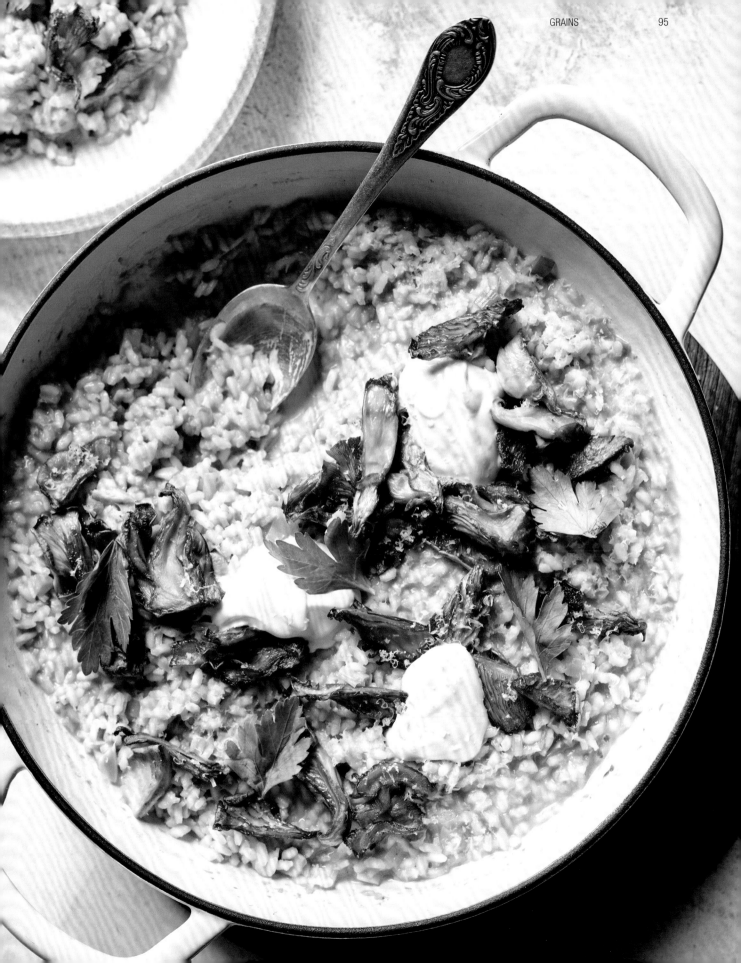

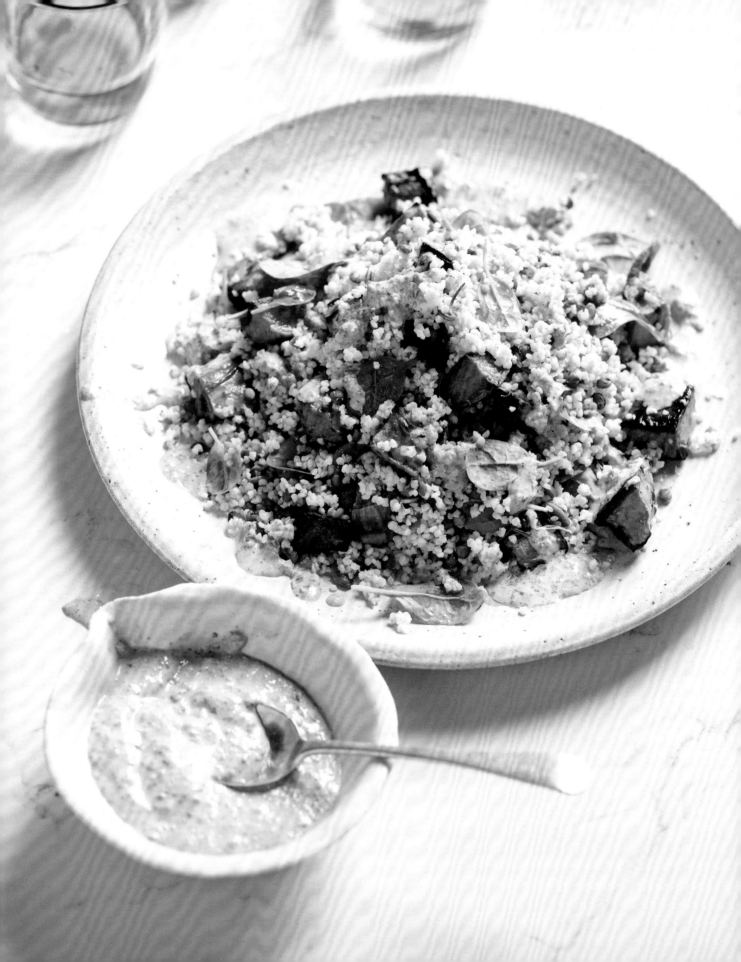

MILLET SALAD WITH PESTO YOGHURT DRESSING

SERVES 4

200g (7oz) sweet potato, cut into 2cm (¾ inch) cubes

1 tsp olive oil

1 sprig fresh rosemary

¾ cup hulled millet

1⅔ cups water

salt to taste

1 cup baby spinach

¼ cup pumpkin seeds

½ cup canned lentils, drained and rinsed

DRESSING

¼ cup low FODMAP basil pesto (see 'basics', page 232)

¼ cup lactose-free yoghurt

1 tbsp lemon juice

1 tbsp tahini

salt and pepper to taste

Energy 1717kJ/410 Calories, Protein 14.1g, Total Fat 20.4g, Saturated Fat 3.4g, Carbohydrate 39.4g, Sugars 5.1g, Dietary fibre 6.2g, Calcium 108mg, Iron 4.7mg.

1. Preheat the oven to 200°C/400°F.

2. Spread the sweet potato on a baking tray lined with baking paper. Drizzle with olive oil and scatter with rosemary leaves. Bake for 20-25 minutes or until golden.

3. Meanwhile, add the millet, water and salt to a saucepan. Bring to the boil then reduce the heat to low and simmer for 15 minutes. Remove the pan from the heat and set aside for 10 minutes. Fluff the mixture with a fork.

4. Transfer the millet to a serving bowl along with the roasted sweet potato, spinach, pumpkin seeds and canned lentils. Stir to combine. Refrigerate for at least an hour before serving.

5. To make the pesto dressing, whisk the dressing ingredients together in a small bowl. Season to taste.

6. Drizzle the dressing over the salad and serve.

SERVING SUGGESTION

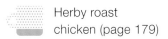
Herby roast chicken (page 179)

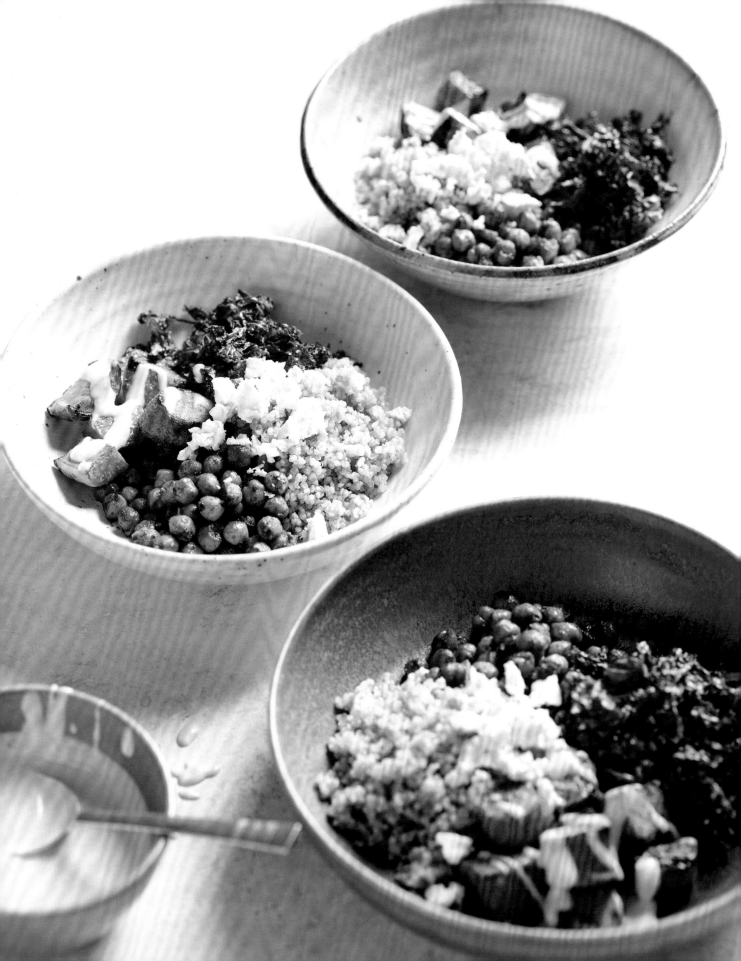

QUINOA BUDDHA BOWL

SERVES 4

300g (10½oz) sweet potato, cut into
   2cm (¾ inch) cubes
2 carrots, roughly chopped
1½ tbsp olive oil
salt and pepper to taste
1 cup kale, chopped
1 cup quinoa
2 cups low FODMAP vegetable stock
1 cup canned chickpeas, drained
   and rinsed
1 tsp smoked paprika
½ tsp chilli flakes (optional)
½ cup fetta, crumbled

DRESSING

¼ cup tahini
1 tbsp maple syrup
half a lemon, juiced
⅓ cup hot water

Energy 2149kJ/514 Caolories, Protein
19.6g, Total Fat 15.5 g, Saturated Fat 4.6g,
Carbohydrate 66.9g, Sugars 24g, Dietary
fibre 14.4g, Calcium 233.8mg, Iron 4.2mg.

1. Preheat the oven to 200°C/400°F. Line a tray with baking paper.

2. Toss the sweet potato and carrot with 1 tbsp of the olive oil and salt and pepper to taste. Place on the tray and roast for 25 minutes or until golden.

3. Add the kale to the oven tray and cook for a further 5 minutes.

4. Meanwhile, add the quinoa and vegetable stock to a small saucepan. Bring to the boil, then lower the heat and simmer, uncovered, until cooked through (approximately 15 minutes).

5. Heat the remaining ½ tbsp of olive oil in a frypan over medium heat, add the chickpeas, paprika and chilli flakes to the pan and cook, stirring, for 3-4 minutes or until heated through. Set aside.

6. To make the tahini dressing, combine the tahini, maple syrup and lemon juice in a small bowl and whisk to combine. Slowly add the hot water and whisk until a pourable sauce forms.

7. To serve, divide the quinoa, sweet potato, carrot, kale and chickpeas among four bowls. Top with fetta and drizzle over the tahini dressing.

POLENTA CHIPS

SERVES 4 (MAKES 24)
400ml (14 fl oz) water
150g (5oz) instant polenta
40g (1½oz) parmesan cheese, shaved
2 tsp dried oregano
olive oil for brushing
sea salt flakes to taste
2 tbsp instant polenta for dusting
'garlic' aioli to serve (see 'basics',
  page 228)

Energy 849kJ/203 Calories, Protein 7.8g,
Total Fat 5.4g, Saturated Fat 2.4g,
Carbohydrate 29.3g, Sugars 0.3g, Dietary
fibre 1.9g, Calcium 119.5mg, Iron 0.8mg.

1. Bring the water to the boil, gradually whisk in the polenta, then stir for 1-2 minutes or until thick.

2. Stir in the parmesan and oregano.

3. Line a baking tray with baking paper. Spread the polenta into the tray. Cover and refrigerate for 1 hour to allow the polenta to firm up.

4. Preheat the oven to 210°C/410°F. Cut the polenta into chips and brush with olive oil. Dust the chips with extra polenta and sprinkle with sea salt flakes to taste.

5. Line a separate baking tray with baking paper, space out the polenta chips on the tray and bake for 30 minutes or until golden. Check the chips after 20 minutes to make sure they do not crisp up too much.

6. Serve warm with 'garlic' aioli for dipping.

SERVING SUGGESTION

 Garlic aioli (page 228)

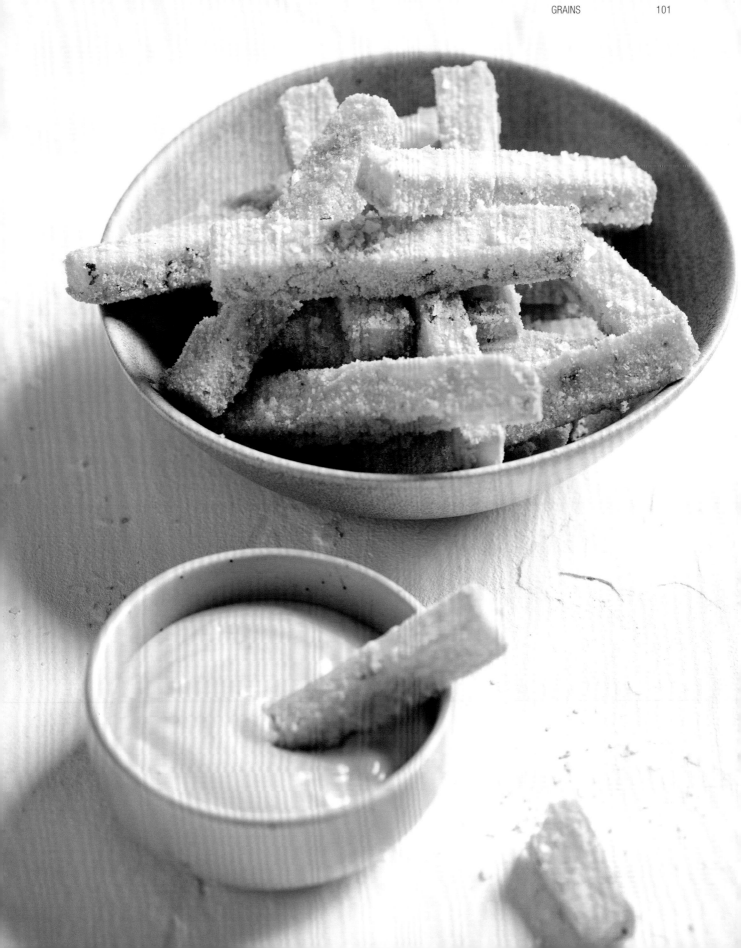

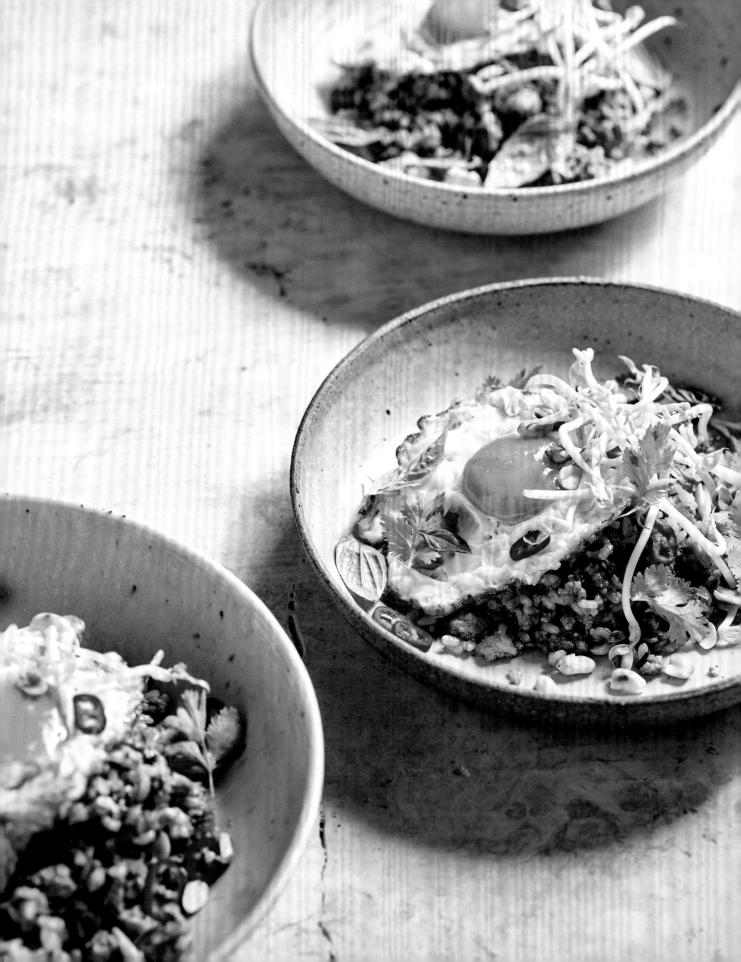

NASI GORENG

SERVES 4

2 tbsp grated ginger

¼ cup spring onions (scallions) (green tops only), thinly sliced

500g (1lb) chicken mince

1 tbsp sesame oil

4 large eggs

1 tbsp garlic-infused olive oil

3 cups cooked brown rice

2 tbsp tamari

¼ cup kecap manis

1 cup bean sprouts

2 long red chillies, finely sliced

½ cup Thai basil leaves, chopped

½ cup coriander leaves, chopped

½ cup peanuts, chopped

Energy 2980kJ/712 Calories, Protein 42.5g, Total Fat 36.5g, Saturated Fat 6.8g, Carbohydrate 62.5g, Sugars 15.5g, Dietary fibre 5.8g, Calcium 87.9mg, Iron 4.2mg.

1. Heat the garlic-infused olive oil in a wok over high heat, then add the ginger, spring onion tops and chicken. Stir-fry for 5 minutes or until the chicken is cooked through. Remove the chicken from the wok and set aside.

2. Add the sesame oil to the wok, then break in the eggs, one at a time. Cook for 2-3 minutes or until done to your taste. Transfer the cooked eggs to a separate dish and keep warm.

3. Add the rice, tamari and kecap manis and stir-fry for 4 minutes.

4. To serve, divide the rice mixture between bowls. Top with the eggs and bean sprouts and sprinkle with chilli, basil, coriander and peanuts.

SERVING SUGGESTION

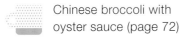

Chinese broccoli with oyster sauce (page 72)

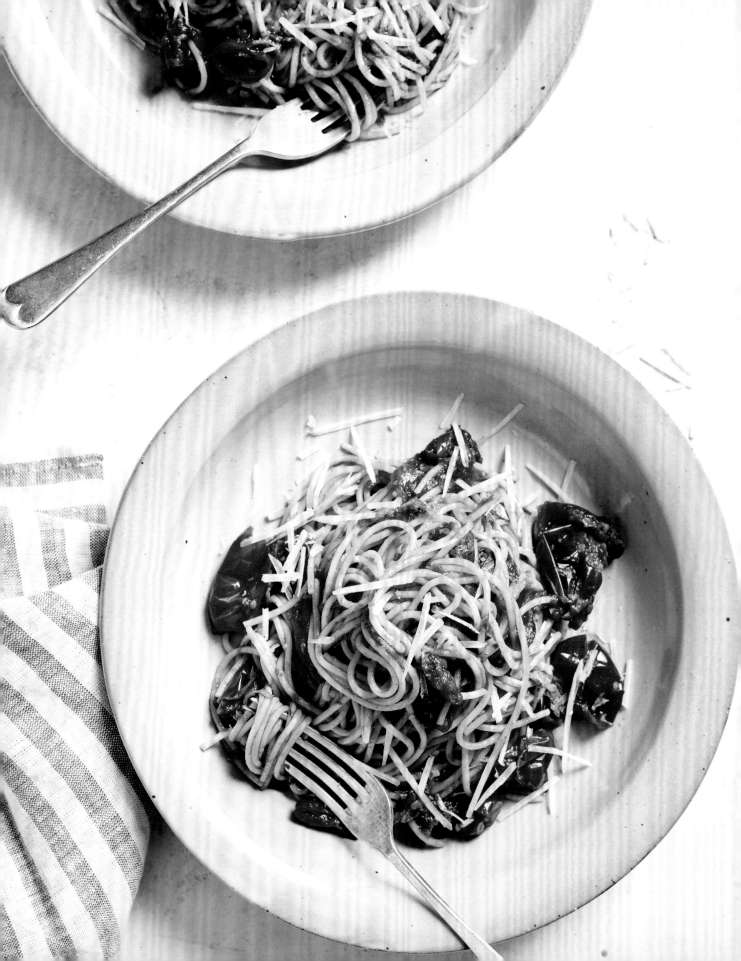

PUTTANESCA

SERVES 4

450g (1lb) truss tomatoes, chopped
   into wedges
2 tbsp garlic-infused olive oil
salt and pepper to taste
1 long red chilli, finely chopped
6 anchovy fillets
1 tbsp capers, chopped
2 tbsp dry white wine
400g (14oz) gluten-free spaghetti
1 lemon, juiced
¼ cup flat-leaved parsley, chopped
40g (1½oz) grated parmesan

Energy 2198.6kJ/526 Calories, Protein
12.5g, Total Fat 14.4g, Saturated Fat 4.2g,
Carbohydrate 80.5g, Sugars 3.3g, Dietary
fibre 5.1g, Calcium 160mg, Iron 2.6g.

1. Preheat the oven to 180°C/350°F.

2. Place the chopped tomatoes on a baking tray and drizzle with 1 tbsp of the garlic-infused olive oil. Season the tomatoes with salt and pepper and roast for 20 minutes or until lightly browned and caramelised.

3. Heat the remaining 1 tbsp of oil in a large frypan over medium heat.

4. Add the chilli and anchovies and cook for 1-2 minutes, stirring until the anchovies melt. Add the capers, white wine and caramelised tomatoes (including cooking juices).

5. Bring the sauce to a simmer and stir for approximately 3 minutes, or until thick and rich. Adjust the seasoning according to taste.

6. Cook the spaghetti in a large pot of salted boiling water until al dente. Drain the pasta well then toss it with the puttanesca sauce.

7. Add the lemon juice and parsley. Serve sprinkled with grated parmesan.

PERSIAN PILAF

SERVES 6

½ tsp saffron threads

¼ cup boiling water, plus 1 cup extra

½ cup pine nuts

2 cups basmati rice

100g (3½oz) dried cranberries

2 tbsp butter

1 cup spring onions (scallions)
   (green tops only), finely chopped

2 medium-sized carrots, chopped
   into matchsticks

1 tsp cinnamon

½ tsp cumin seeds, ground

½ tsp cardamom, ground

½ tsp cloves, ground

¼ tsp turmeric

salt and pepper to taste

Energy 1884 kJ/450 Calories, Protein
7.6g, Total Fat 15.6g, Saturated Fat 2.7g,
Carbohydrate 67.8g, Sugars 15.8g, Dietary
fibre 4.8g, Calcium 24.3mg, Iron 1.0mg.

1. Place the saffron threads in a bowl with the boiling water and
    set aside to infuse for 10 minutes. Meanwhile, toast the pine
    nuts in a small pan over medium heat for 3 minutes or until they
    begin to brown. Transfer to a plate and set aside to cool.

2. Rinse the rice well under cold running water. Cook the rice in
    a pot of salted boiling water for approximately 6 minutes or
    until al dente. Drain rice if needed. Set aside.

3. Place the cranberries in a small bowl with the remaining 1 cup
    boiling water and set aside for five minutes, then drain.

4. Heat the butter in a large frypan over medium heat. Add in
    the spring onion (scallion) tops, carrots, and spices and stir
    until fragrant.

5. Stir in the saffron water, rice and cranberries, cover and cook
    for 5 minutes or until all the liquid has been absorbed.
    Scatter with the pine nuts and serve.

SERVING SUGGESTION

 Middle Eastern
fish with tahini
sauce (page 158)

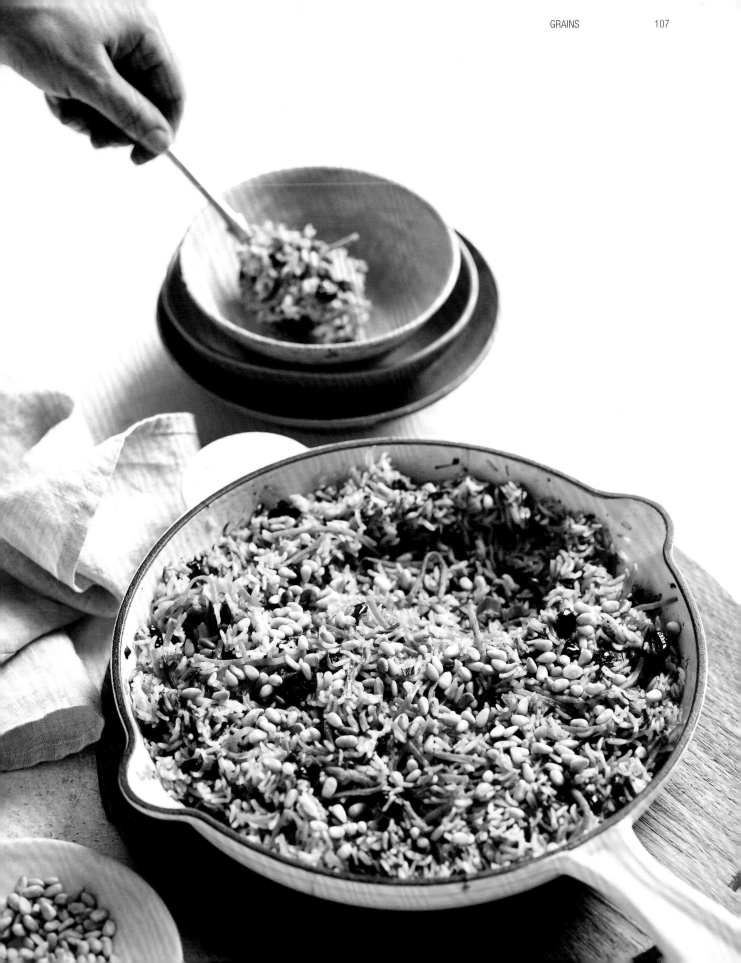

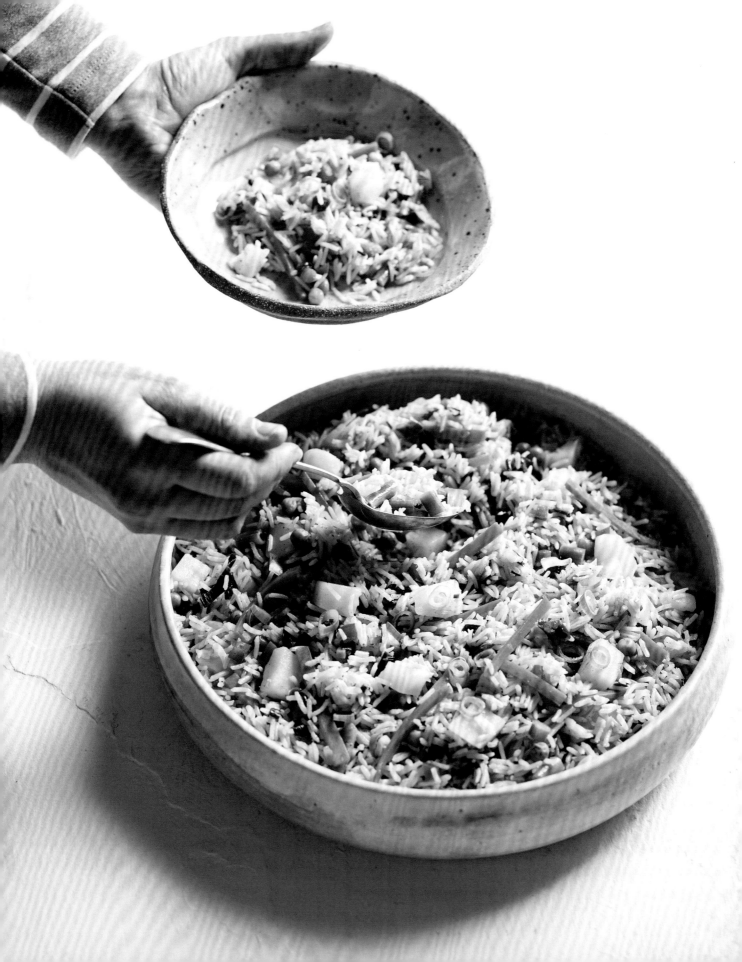

INDIAN RICE WITH VEGETABLES

SERVES 6

1 tbsp garlic-infused olive oil

1 cup spring onions (scallions) (green tops only), finely chopped

2 cups long grain white rice

4 cups hot water

1 tsp salt, or to taste

1 tsp garam marsala

2 small carrots, cut into matchstick

60g (2oz) green beans, thinly sliced

½ cup red capsicum (bell pepper), diced

1 small potato, peeled and cut into cubes

½ cup green peas, fresh or frozen

Energy 1292kJ/309 Calories, Protein 7g, Total Fat 3.9g, Saturated Fat 0.6g, Carbohydrate 59.2g, Sugars 3.0g, Dietary fibre 3.0g, Calcium 22.1mg, Iron 0.6mg.

1. Preheat a heavy-based casserole dish with a tight fitting lid over low heat. Add the garlic-infused olive oil add spring onion (scallion) tops and cook for 5 minutes, stirring occasionally.

2. Add the rice and cook for 2-3 minutes, stirring occasionally. Add the hot water, salt and garam masala, increase the heat and bring the mixture to the boil, then turn the heat to very low. Cover the dish with a tight fitting lid and cook for 10 minutes.

3. Top the rice with the carrot sticks, sliced green beans, red capsicum, potato cubes and green beans (do not stir the vegetables into the rice). Sprinkle with salt to taste. Cover and cook over very low heat for 10-15 minutes or until the vegetables are cooked.

4. Gently stir the vegetables through the rice (the rice should be fluffy). Serve immediately.

SERVING SUGGESTION

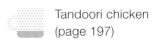
Tandoori chicken (page 197)

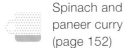
Spinach and paneer curry (page 152)

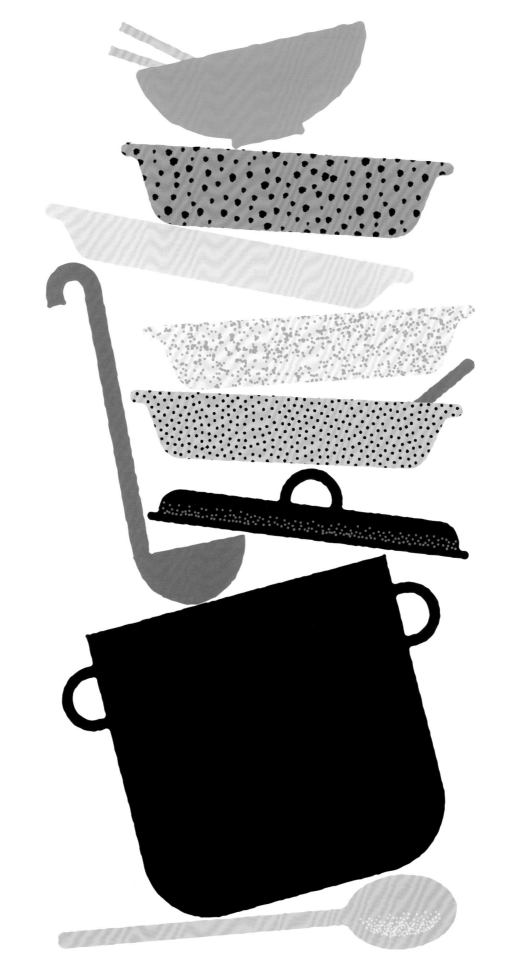

SOUPS

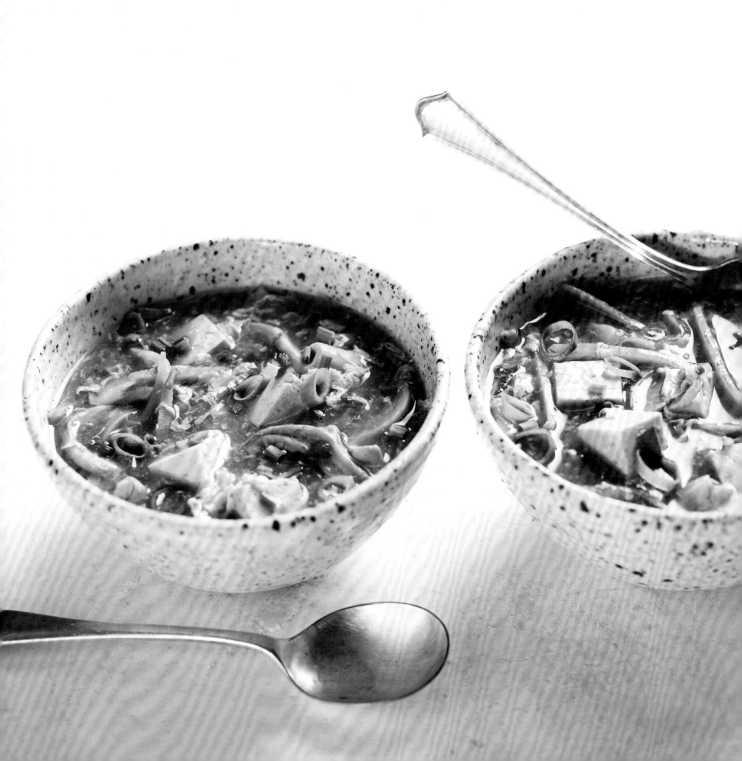

HOT AND SOUR SOUP

SERVES 4

1 tbsp garlic-infused olive oil

2 large red chillies, deseeded and
   roughly chopped

1 tbsp finely grated ginger

salt and pepper to taste

6 cups low FODMAP vegetable stock

1 tbsp vegetable oil

250g (9oz) oyster mushrooms,
   roughly torn

225g (8oz) bamboo shoots, finely sliced

2 tbsp soy sauce

¼ cup rice wine vinegar

1 tsp maple syrup

300g (10½oz) firm tofu, cubed

2 medium-sized carrots, chopped
   into matchsticks

2 tbsp cornflour (cornstarch)

1 tbsp water

2 large eggs, whisked

¼ cup chives, roughly chopped

¼ cup spring onions (scallions) (green
   tops only), roughly chopped

Energy 1235kJ/295 Calories, Protein
16.1g, Total Fat 17.8g, Saturated Fat 2.9g,
Carbohydrate 12.0g, Sugars 6.0g, Dietary
fibre 8.4g, Calcium 298.2mg, Iron 3.8mg.

1. Place the garlic-infused olive oil, roughly chopped red chillies and ginger into either a mortar and pestle or small food processor. Add the salt and pepper and blitz or pound until a rough paste forms.

2. Place the low FODMAP vegetable stock in a pot over low heat.

3. Heat the vegetable oil in a wok over medium-high heat. Add the mushrooms and stir-fry for 3-4 minutes.
   Add the pre-prepared chilli paste and bamboo shoots and cook for an additional minute.

4. Mix the soy sauce, rice wine vinegar and maple syrup in a bowl or jug. Add the mixture to the wok and cook for approximately 1 minute. Pour in the hot vegetable stock and bring to the boil. Reduce to a simmer and cook for 10 minutes.

5. Add in the tofu and carrots to the wok and cook for 1 minute. Meanwhile, place the cornflour and water into a small bowl and stir until the mixture forms a slurry. Add the mixture to the wok and stir continuously for 30 seconds.

6. Slowly stir the whisked eggs into the soup. Serve garnished with chives and spring onion (scallion) tops.

MISO SOUP

SERVES 4

4 tbsp miso paste

2 cups low FODMAP vegetable stock

1 tbsp mirin

¼ cup spring onions (scallions)
    (green tops only)

1 tbsp wakame, thinly sliced

1 tsp finely grated lemon zest

200g (7oz) firm tofu, cut into
    bite-sized cubes

1 tbsp toasted sesame seeds

1. Add the miso paste, stock and mirin to a saucepan and bring to the boil.

2. Add half the spring onion (scallion) tops and set the rest aside.

3. Stir in the wakame flakes, reduce the heat to low and simmer for 1-2 minutes. Stir in the lemon zest.

4. Divide the tofu between four small bowls. Pour the soup over the tofu and garnish with the remaining spring onion and sesame seeds.

5. Serve immediately.

Energy 583kJ/139 Calories, Protein 10.0g,
Total Fat 6.6g, Saturated Fat 0.9g,
Carbohydrate 7.7g, Sugars 4.7g, Dietary
fibre 3.2g, Calcium 185.0mg, Iron 2.1mg.

SERVING SUGGESTION

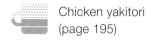 Chicken yakitori
(page 195)

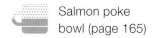 Salmon poke
bowl (page 165)

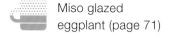 Miso glazed
eggplant (page 71)

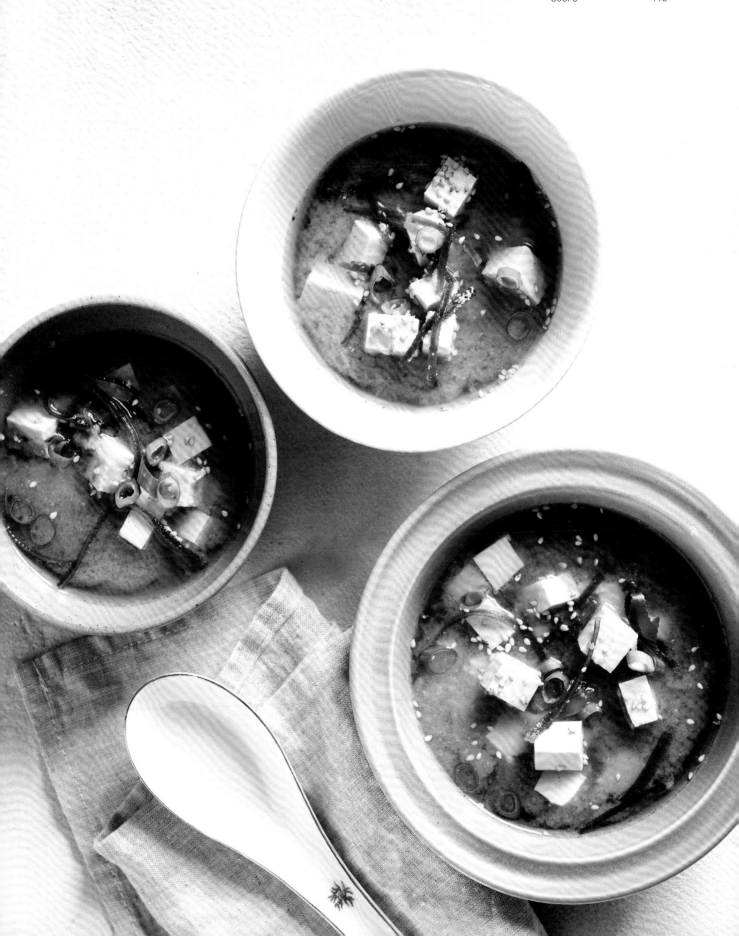

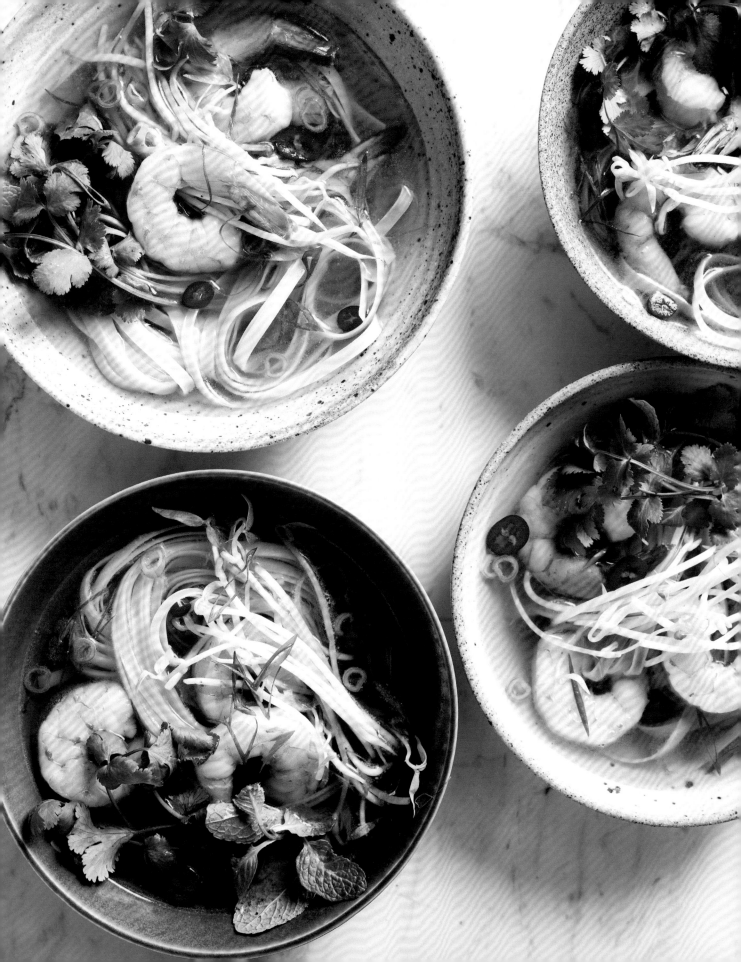

PRAWN PHO

SERVES 4

50g (2oz) ginger, peeled and sliced

2 star anise, whole

1 tbsp soy sauce

1 tbsp fish sauce

2 cups water

400g (14oz) green prawns, peeled
and deveined

4 cups low FODMAP chicken stock

150g (5oz) pad Thai rice noodles

100g (3½oz) bean shoots

¼ cup mint leaves

¼ cup coriander (cilantro)

¼ cup spring onions (scallions) (green
tops only), finely sliced

1 large red chilli, finely sliced

Energy 1260 kJ/301 Calories, Protein
27.0g, Total Fat 1.3g, Saturated Fat 0.4g,
Carbohydrate 42.0g, Sugars 1.8g, Dietary
fibre 3.3g, Calcium 178.6mg, Iron 2.4mg.

1. In a large saucepan, combine the ginger, star anise, soy sauce, fish sauce and water, and bring to the boil over high heat.

2. Add the prawns and reduce the heat to medium. Simmer the prawns until they change colour; this should take approximately 4 minutes.

3. Remove the ginger and star anise (discard). Remove the prawns with a slotted spoon and set aside on a plate. Return the liquid to a simmer and add the chicken stock. Leave the liquid to simmer again.

4. Place the noodles in a heatproof bowl and pour in enough boiling water to cover them. Set aside for 5 minutes to soften, then drain and divide between serving bowls.

5. To serve, divide the stock mixture between bowls. Garnish with the cooked prawns, bean shoots, herbs, spring onion (scallion) tops and chilli.

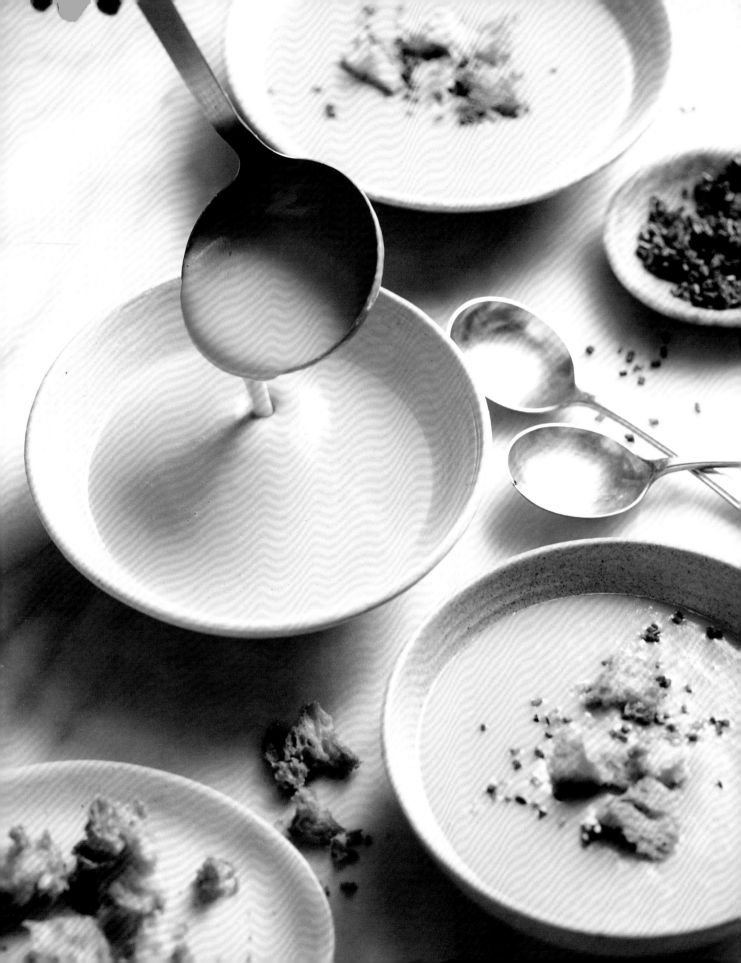

LEEK AND POTATO SOUP

SERVES 4

2 tbsp garlic-infused olive oil

1 cup finely chopped spring onions
(scallions) (green tops only)

4 cups coarsely chopped leek
(green tops only)

4 medium-sized potatoes, peeled
and diced

¼ tsp thyme leaves

5 cups low FODMAP chicken stock

100g (3½oz) low FODMAP sourdough
bread, chopped into large cubes

2 tbsp olive oil

ground black pepper and salt to taste

2 tbsp chives, finely chopped

Energy 1547kJ/370 Calories, Protein
8.3g, Total Fat 20.2g, Saturated Fat 3.3g,
Carbohydrate 35.3g, Sugars 4.6 g, Dietary
fibre 4.8 g, Calcium 55.0mg, Iron 2.0mg.

1. Preheat a large heavy-based saucepan over medium heat.

2. Add the oil, and when hot, add the spring onion tops (scallions).
Cook for 2-3 minutes until soft.

3. Stir in the chopped leek, diced potatoes and thyme leaves.
Cook while stirring for 3 minutes.

4. Pour in the chicken stock and bring to the boil, reduce the heat
to medium and simmer for approximately 20 minutes or until
the potatoes are well cooked. Cool slightly, then blitz in batches
in a food processor until smooth, transferring each batch to a
clean saucepan. Set aside.

5. To make the low FODMAP croutons, preheat the oven to
200°C/400°F. Spread the bread cubes on a baking tray and
pour over the oil. Toss to coat each bread cube in oil and bake
for 10-15 minutes or until the croutons are golden and crisp.

6. Reheat the soup over medium heat, adding salt and ground
black pepper to taste. Serve topped with a sprinkle of chives
and low FODMAP croutons.

MISO CHICKEN RAMEN

SERVES 4

500g (1lb) chicken breast

salt and pepper to taste

1 tbsp garlic-infused olive oil

1 tbsp sesame oil

1 tbsp finely grated ginger

⅓ cup soy sauce

⅓ cup mirin

¼ cup miso paste

1 tbsp white sugar

8 cups low FODMAP chicken stock

180g (6oz) bok choy, leaves separated (2 bunches)

2 cups oyster mushrooms

250g (9oz) rice noodles

4 large eggs, soft-boiled, peeled and halved lengthways

¼ cup spring onions (scallions) (green tops only), finely sliced

1 tbsp sesame seeds, toasted

Energy 3014kJ/720 Calories, Protein 47.9g, Total Fat 17.6g, Saturated Fat 3.8g, Carbohydrate 84.2g, Sugars 15.7g, Dietary fibre 5.0g, Calcium 152.0mg, Iron 4.1mg.

1. Preheat the oven to 180°C/350°F.

2. Season the chicken with salt and pepper to taste. Add the garlic-infused olive oil to a large, oven-safe pan over medium heat.

3. Add the chicken to the pan and cook for 5 minutes on each side or until golden brown. Transfer the pan to the oven and roast for 15-20 minutes or until the chicken is cooked through. Remove the chicken from the oven, transfer to a plate and cover with foil until ready to serve.

4. Add the sesame oil and ginger to the pan and cook over medium heat 1-2 minutes until softened.

5. Add the soy sauce, mirin, miso paste and sugar and stir to dissolve the sugar.

6. Add the stock, cover the pan with a lid and bring to the boil. Remove the lid, reduce the heat to medium and simmer for 5 minutes.

7. Add the bok choy and oyster mushrooms and simmer for a few minutes or until the bok choy is wilted. Season with salt to taste.

8. Meanwhile, cook the noodles according to packet instructions. Once cooked, divide the noodles evenly between four bowls.

9. Slice the chicken into thin pieces and divide it between the serving bowls along with the ramen broth and vegetables. Top the ramen with thinly sliced spring onion tops (scallions) and eggs and scatter with sesame seeds. Serve immediately.

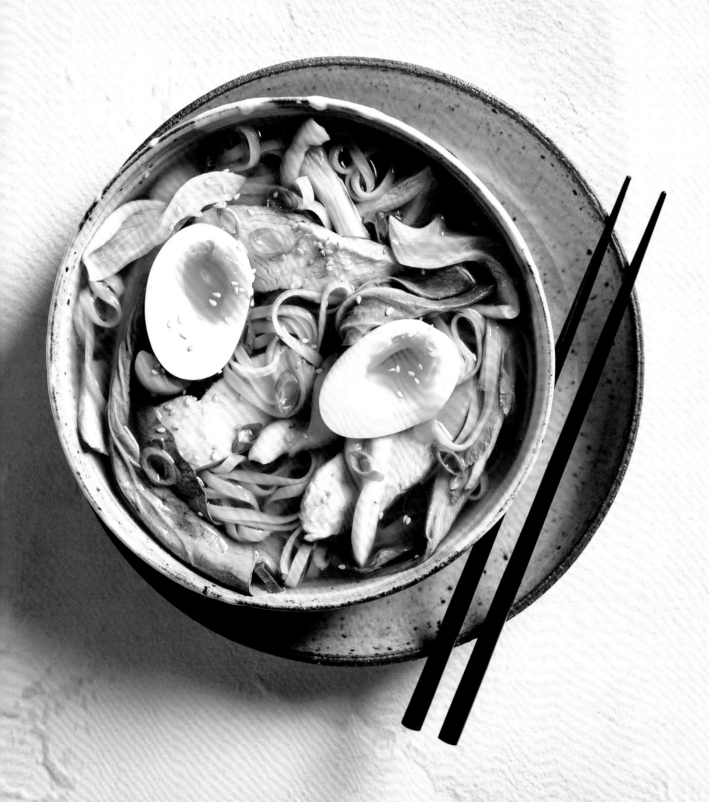

ROASTED PUMPKIN AND CARROT SOUP

SERVES 6

1kg (2lb 2oz) kent pumpkin (squash), peeled and cut into 1cm (½ inch) pieces

800g (1lb 8oz) carrots, peeled and cut into 1cm (½ inch) pieces

2 tbsp garlic-infused olive oil

2 tbsp olive oil

2 tsp ground coriander

1 tsp ground cumin

1 tsp ground turmeric

½ tsp ground cardamom

½ tsp paprika

¼ tsp chilli powder (optional)

4 cups low FODMAP vegetable stock

2 cups water

2 tbsp coriander (cilantro) leaves

Energy 887kJ/212 Calories, Protein 2.6g, Total Fat 12.9g, Saturated Fat 2.1g, Carbohydrate 17.2g, Sugars 15.7g, Dietary fibre 7.5g, Calcium 73.8mg, Iron 1.2mg.

1. Preheat the oven to 210°C/410°F.

2. Place the pumpkin (squash) and carrot on a tray lined with baking paper and drizzle over 1 tbsp of the garlic-infused oil and 1 tbsp of the olive oil. Toss to coat. Bake for 30-35 minutes or until golden brown.

3. Meanwhile, heat the remaining oils in a large saucepan over medium heat. Add the spices and cook while stirring for 1-2 minutes or until aromatic.

4. Increase the heat to high and add the roasted carrot and pumpkin as well as the stock and water. Cover and bring to the boil. Reduce the heat to low and simmer for 15 minutes.

5. Remove from heat. Using a stick mixer, blend the soup until smooth. Serve hot garnished with coriander.

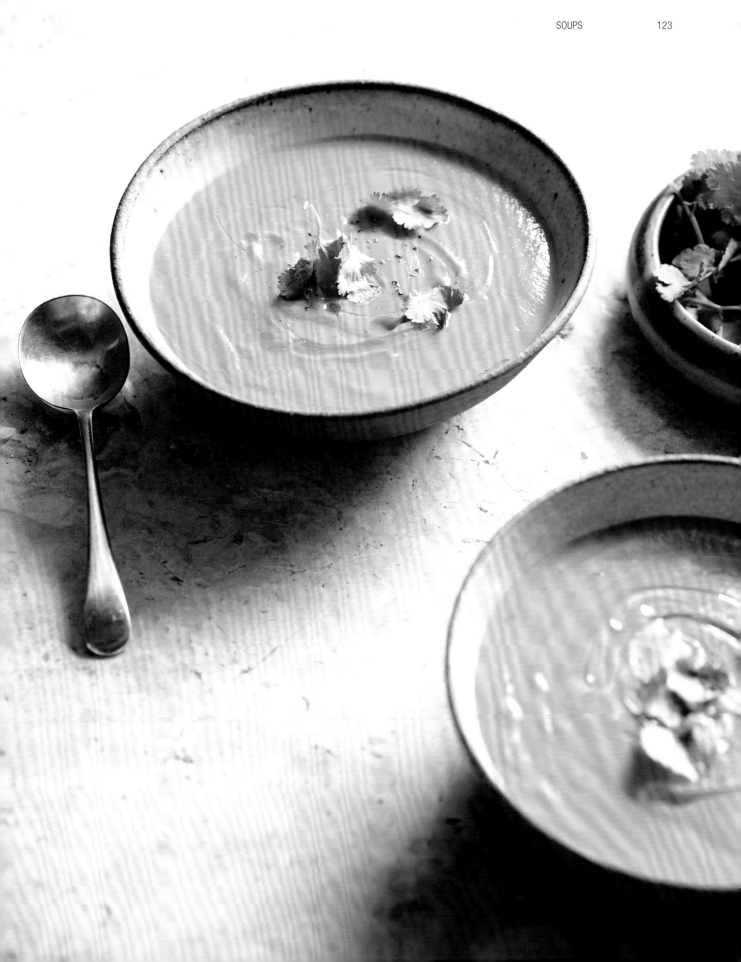

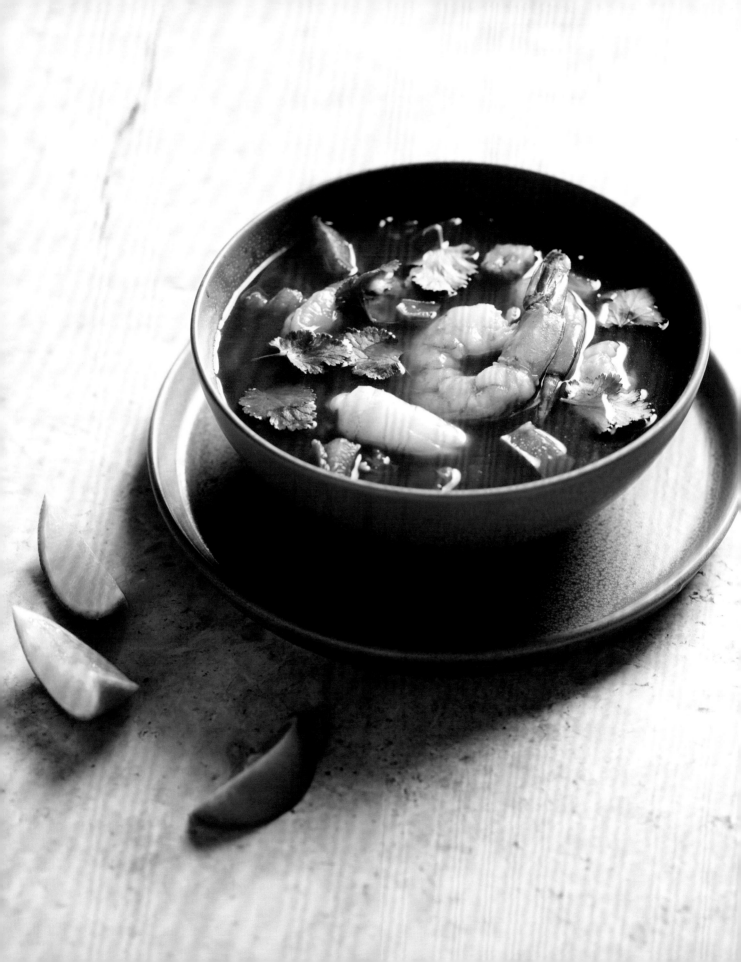

TOM YUM SOUP

SERVES 4

2½ cm (1 inch) piece galangal, peeled
  and thinly sliced

2 lemongrass stalks, bruised

5 small red chillies, coarsely chopped

3 tbsp tomato paste

1 cup coriander (cilantro) (including
  stalks and roots), coarsely chopped

8 makrut (kaffir) lime leaves

4 cups low FODMAP chicken stock

400g (14oz) green prawns, peeled
  and deveined

2 Roma tomatoes, diced

3 tsp sugar

¼ cup fish sauce

¼ cup lime juice

coriander (cilantro) leaves to serve

lime wedges to serve

Energy 635kJ/152 Calories, Protein 23.9g,
Total Fat 1.3g, Saturated Fat 0.4g,
Carbohydrate 8.9g, Sugars 7.7g, Dietary
fibre 2.7g, Calcium 162.4mg, Iron 2.3mg.

1. Place the galangal, lemongrass, chillies, tomato paste, coriander (cilantro) and lime leaves and stock in a large saucepan over high heat and bring to the boil.

2. Reduce the heat to medium and simmer uncovered for 20 minutes.

3. Strain the soup through a fine sieve, discard the solids and return the liquid to the pan.

4. Reheat the soup until it starts to simmer, then add the prawns, tomatoes, sugar, fish sauce and lime juice to the pan. Simmer for a further 2 minutes.

5. Serve the soup garnished with coriander leaves and a lime wedge.

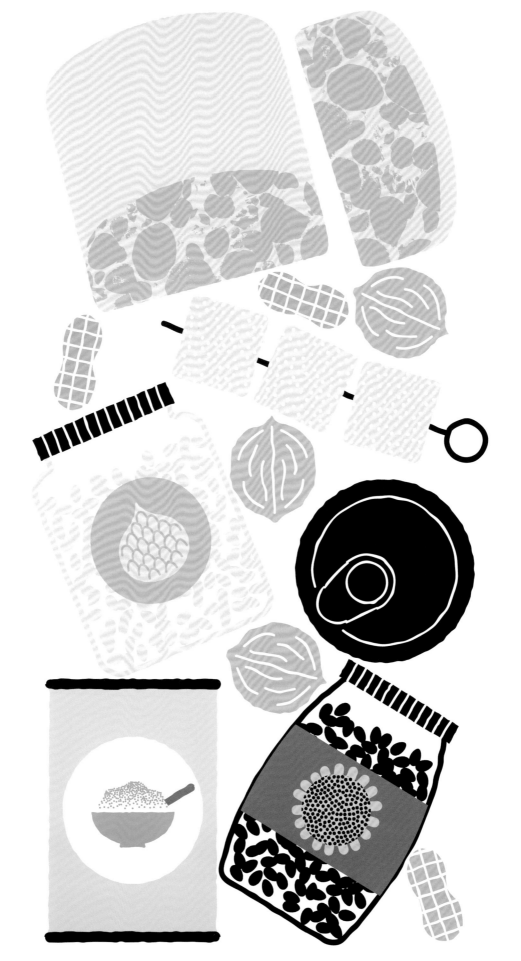

VEGETARIAN AND VEGAN MAINS

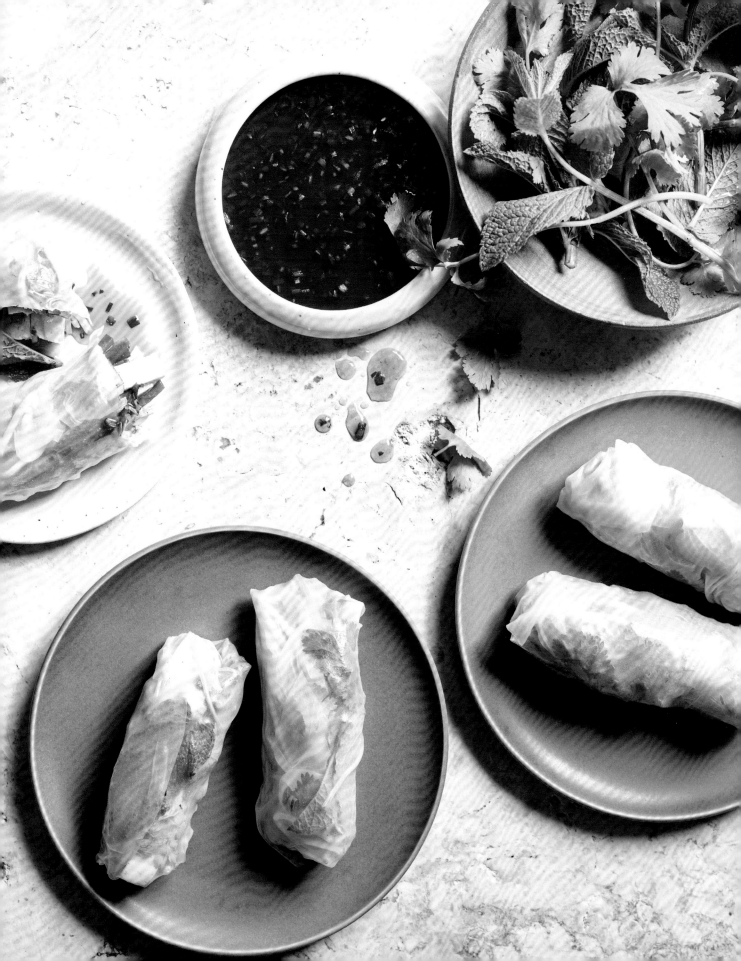

VIETNAMESE RICE PAPER ROLLS

SERVES 6

1 tbsp peanut oil

340g (12oz) firm tofu

24 rice paper wrappers

1 medium-sized red capsicum (bell pepper), thinly sliced

1¼ cup bean sprouts

1 cup mint leaves, firmly packed

1 cup coriander (cilantro) leaves, firmly packed

DIPPING SAUCE

2 tbsp low FODMAP vegan fish sauce

¼ cup lime juice

¼ cup palm sugar

¼ cup low FODMAP vegan oyster sauce

1 small red chilli, finely chopped

Energy 1405kJ/336 Calories, Protein 15.7g, Total Fat 8.6g, Saturated Fat 1.2g, Carbohydrate 46.7g, Sugars 10.4g, Dietary fibre 6.3g, Calcium 245.5mg, Iron 4.0mg.

1. To make the dipping sauce, whisk all the ingredients in a small saucepan over medium heat until the sugar dissolves. Transfer to a serving dish and set aside in the refrigerator.

2. Heat the oil in a small frypan and brown the tofu on both sides. Cut into 24 thin slices and set aside.

3. Working in batches, soak the rice paper in a bowl of warm water until softened. Place on a work surface and pat dry with paper towel. Arrange a portion of the tofu, capsicum, bean sprouts and herbs in a line along the centre of each wrapper. Fold the left and right sides in towards the centre, then roll up from bottom to top to enclose the filling. Repeat the process with the remaining ingredients. Refrigerate until ready to serve.

4. Serve the rolls chilled with the dipping sauce.

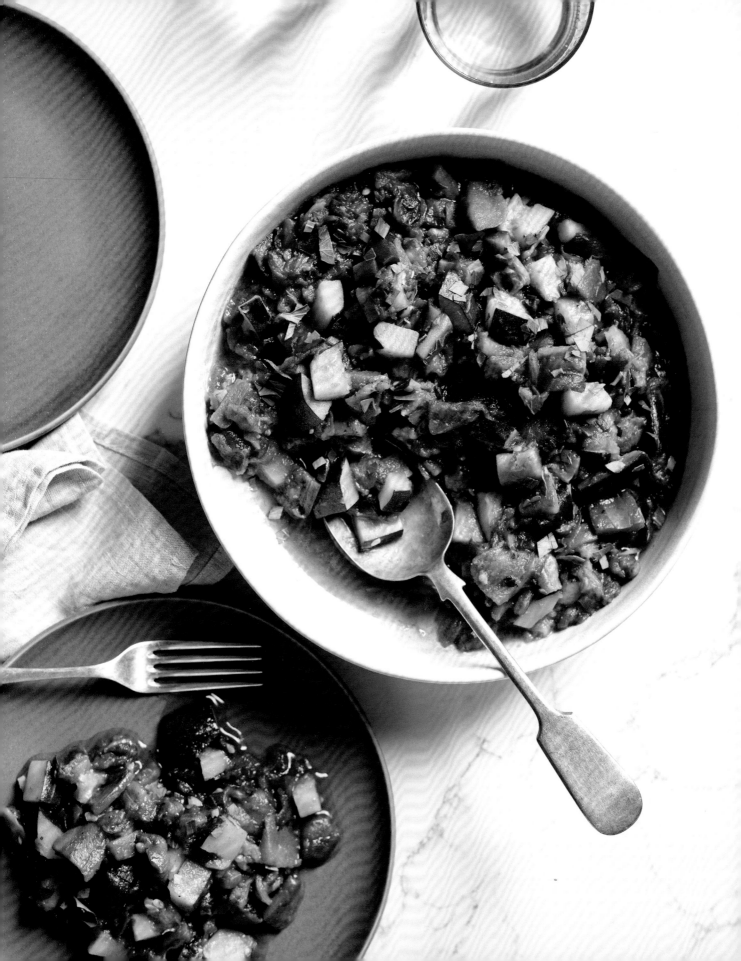

RATATOUILLE

SERVES 6

1 large or 2 small eggplants
(aubergine) (450g/1lb), sliced 1cm
(⅜ inch) thick

salt to taste

olive oil for frying

1 cup spring onions (scallions) (green
tops only), finely chopped

200g (7oz) red capsicum (bell pepper),
chargrilled, peeled and seeded

200g (7oz) green capsicum
(bell pepper), chargrilled, peeled
and seeded

1 zucchini (courgette), chopped

4 tomatoes (common/truss), peeled,
seeded and chopped

6 coriander seeds, crushed

¼ tsp black pepper, freshly ground

2 tbsp parsley, finely chopped

Energy 216.2kJ/52 Calories, Protein
2.7g, Total Fat 0.5g, Saturated Fat 0g,
Carbohydrate 6.8g, Sugars 6.5g, Dietary
fibre 4.3g, Calcium 39.8mg, Iron 0.8mg.

1. Spread the eggplant (aubergine) on a tray and sprinkle with salt. Place absorbent paper over the eggplant and set aside for 1 hour to allow the paper to absorb the juices.

2. Rinse the salt off the eggplant and dry with absorbent paper. Chop the eggplant into cubes and set aside.

3. Heat a heavy-based casserole (with a well-fitted lid) over medium heat. Add the oil, then add the chopped spring onion (scallion) tops, reduce the heat to low and cook for 3-5 minutes or until softened.

4. Add the chopped capsicums (bell peppers) and eggplant to the casserole dish and stir. Cover with the lid and cook over low heat for 40 minutes, stirring occasionally.

5. Add the chopped zucchini (courgette), chopped tomato, crushed coriander and freshly ground pepper. Stir well and cook over low heat for a further 30 minutes or until the vegetables are tender.

6. Sprinkle with freshly chopped parsley and stir well. Adjust seasoning to taste and serve.

GREEN FALAFELS

SERVES 5

300g (10½oz) English spinach
1 cup parsley
½ cup mint
¼ cup spring onions (scallions)
(green tops only)
½ cup walnuts
1 cup white quinoa, cooked
1 cup canned chickpeas, drained
2 tbsp tahini
1 tbsp lemon juice
1 tsp chilli
1 egg
1 tsp cumin
1 tbsp gluten-free flour
½ tsp baking powder
salt and pepper to taste
vegetable oil (for shallow frying)

Energy 1136 kJ/272 Calories, Protein
10.3g, Total Fat 17.3g, Saturated Fat 1.6g,
Carbohydrate 14.9g, Sugars 1.8g, Dietary
fibre 7.6g, Calcium 123.8mg, Iron 4.7mg.

1. Preheat the oven to 200°C/350°F. Line a baking tray with baking paper.

2. Place the spinach, herbs, spring onion (scallion) tops and walnuts in a food processor and pulse until finely chopped.

3. Add the quinoa, chickpeas, tahini, lemon juice, chilli, egg and cumin to the food processor and pulse until well combined.

4. Transfer the mixture to a large bowl. Add the flour and baking powder and mix until well combined. Set aside in the refrigerator for 30 minutes.

5. Shape the mixture into walnut-sized balls.

6. Pour the vegetable oil into a large deep-sided frying pan or saucepan to a depth of 2.5cm (1 inch). Heat over medium-high heat until the oil begins to shimmer. Add the falafels in batches and cook for 3-5 minutes or until crisp on the outside. Remove with a slotted spoon and drain well on paper towels, then transfer to the lined baking tray.

7. Bake for 10-15 minutes, then serve hot.

SERVING SUGGESTION

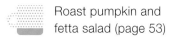

Roast pumpkin and
fetta salad (page 53)

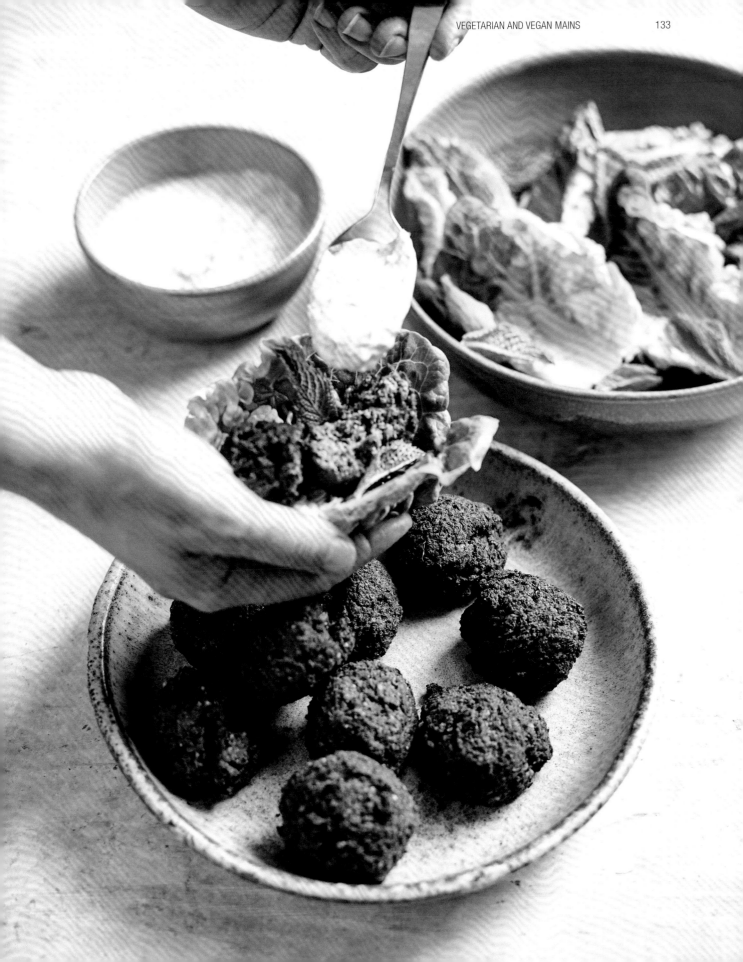

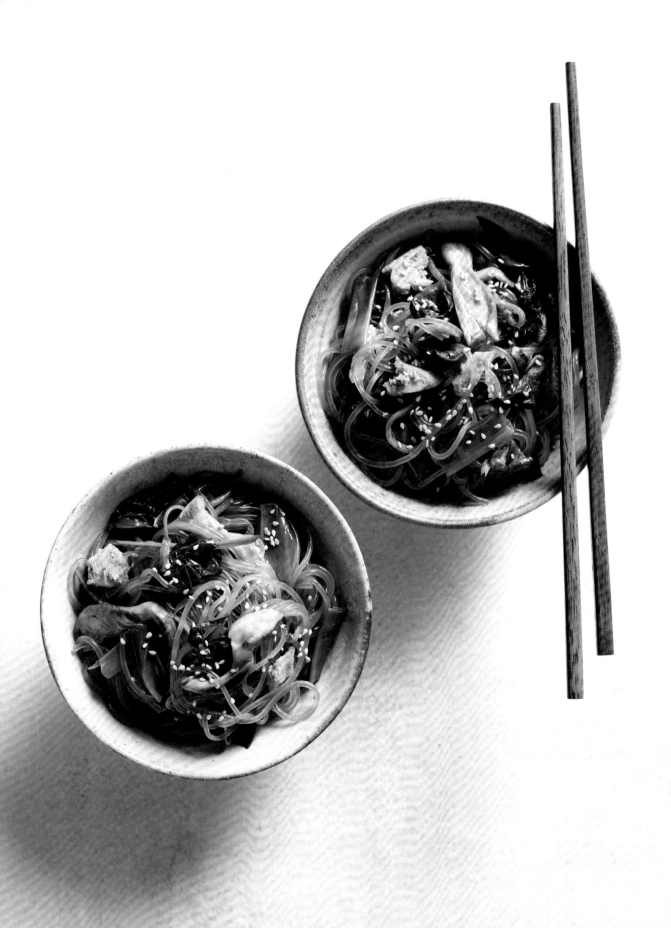

KOREAN GLASS NOODLE STIR-FRY

SERVES 2

125g (4oz) sweet potato noodles (Korean glass noodles)

¼ cup soy sauce

1 tbsp mirin

1 tsp gochugaru (Korean red chilli powder)

1 tsp sesame oil

2 eggs

3 tsp garlic-infused olive oil

150g (5oz) oyster mushrooms, separated into small clumps

1 medium-sized carrot, peeled and sliced into matchsticks

½ cup spring onions (scallions) (green tops only), cut into 2½cm (1 inch) lengths

250g (9oz) spinach, stems trimmed, roughly sliced (1 small bunch)

1 tsp sesame seeds, toasted

Energy 2208kJ/528 Calories, Protein 14.3g, Total Fat 20.9g, Saturated Fat 3.8g, Carbohydrate 63.3g, Sugars 9.6g, Dietary fibre 8.7g, Calcium 172.1mg, Iron 4.4mg.

1. Cook the noodles in a pot of boiling water for 6–8 minutes, or until tender. Drain the noodles and refresh in cold water before draining again. Set aside.

2. In a mixing bowl, combine the soy sauce, mirin, gochugaru and sesame oil.

3. In a separate bowl, whisk the eggs with 2 tbsp of the soy mixture.

4. Heat a wok over medium heat, add 1 tsp of the garlic-infused olive oil, and tilt the wok to coat the base evenly. Add the eggs and cook for 1 minute or until cooked through, turning once. Slice the omelette thinly and set aside.

5. Add 1 tsp of the garlic-infused olive oil to the wok and increase the heat to high. Stir in the mushrooms and cook for 3–4 minutes, or until brown and soft. Remove the mushrooms from the wok.

6. Add another teaspoon of the garlic-infused olive oil to the wok, add the carrots and stir-fry for 1 minute. Add the spring onion (scallion) tops and stir-fry for another minute. Add the remaining soy mixture and bring to the boil.

7. Add the spinach and cook until wilted. Reduce the heat to medium and mix in the noodles and cooked mushrooms. Cook for 1–2 minutes or until the noodles are heated through.

8. To serve, divide the noodles between serving bowls and garnish with the egg and sesame seeds.

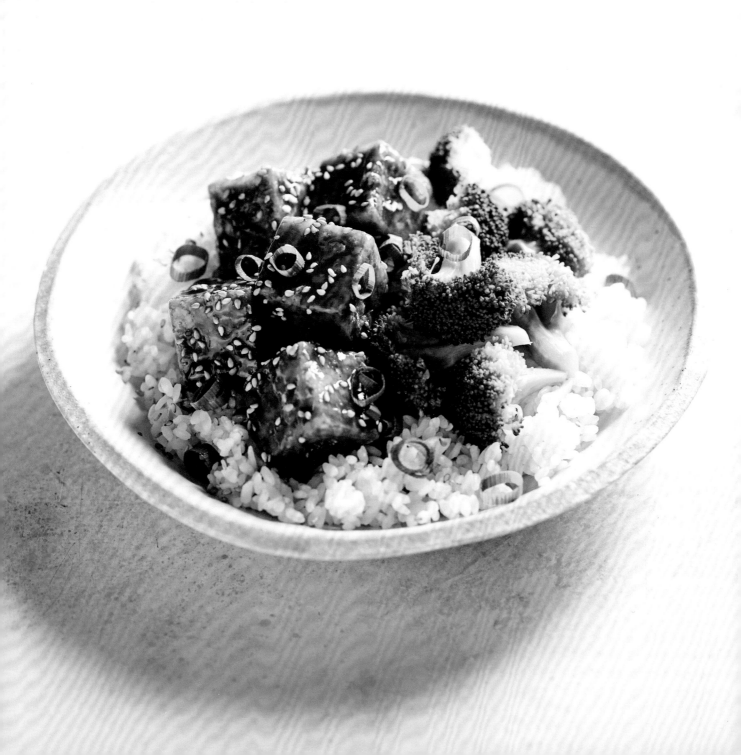

TERIYAKI TOFU BOWLS

SERVES 4

600g (1lb 3oz) firm tofu

2 tbsp cornflour (cornstarch)

1½ cups white rice

300g (10½oz) broccoli heads

1 tbsp garlic-infused olive oil

¼ cup spring onions (scallions) (green tops only) to serve, sliced

1 tbsp sesame seeds to serve

SAUCE

¼ cup soy sauce

¼ cup brown sugar

¼ cup rice wine vinegar

2 tbsp mirin

1 tbsp sesame oil

½ tbsp grated ginger

Energy 2789kJ/667 Calories, Protein 29.1g, Total Fat 22.7g, Saturated Fat 3.2g, Carbohydrate 78.9g, Sugars 13.6g, Dietary fibre 9.3g, Calcium 526.0mg, Iron 5.7mg.

1. Dry the tofu using a paper towel and cut into cubes. Transfer the tofu to a bowl and toss gently to coat with cornflour (cornstarch). Set aside.

2. Cook the rice according to packet instructions and set aside.

3. Meanwhile, cut the broccoli into bite-sized pieces and steam over boiling water until tender.

4. Whisk together all sauce ingredients in a small bowl. Set aside.

5. Heat the garlic-infused olive oil in a large pan over medium heat, add the tofu to the pan and cook, turning occasionally, until lightly browned and crisp.

6. Pour the sauce into the pan and stir until the sauce thickens and forms a shiny glaze; this should take approximately 2–3 minutes.

7. Remove from the heat and divide the tofu, broccoli and rice between four bowls. Sprinkle with spring onion (scallion) tops and sesame seeds to serve.

INDIAN CHANNA DAHL

SERVES 6

⅔ cup channa dahl (split chickpeas)
450ml (1pt) water
¼ cup canola oil
2 tsp black mustard seeds
60 fresh curry leaves
1½ cups finely chopped leek
    (green tops only)
2 tbsp finely grated ginger
1 tsp dried chillies, crushed
3 tsp Madras curry powder
1½ tsp turmeric powder
1 tsp salt
1 small tomato (common/truss),
    finely chopped
2 eggplants (aubergines), diced into
    1cm (½ inch) cubes
¼ cup water
3 cups kale leaves, chopped
1½ tbsp coconut milk powder
¾ cup coriander (cilantro) leaves,
    chopped

Energy 710kJ/170 Calories, Protein 5.0g,
Total Fat 11.9g, Saturated Fat 2.1g,
Carbohydrate 8.3g, sugars 3.3 g, Dietary
fibre 7.3g, Calcium 108.5mg, Iron 3.4mg.

1. Soak the channa dahl in a saucepan of cold water overnight, then drain and rinse. This will reduce the FODMAP content of the channa dahl.

2. Return the channa dal to the sauceapan, add 1½ cups cold water and bring to the boil over high heat. Reduce the heat to low and simmer for 40–50 minutes or until tender, adding extra water if necessary. (Alternatively, cook the soaked channa dahl in a pressure cooker for 20–30 minutes.) Drain and set aside.

3. Heat the oil in a heavy-based saucepan over low heat and add the mustard seeds, curry leaves, leek tops and ginger. Fry for 5 minutes. Take care not to burn.

4. Add the crushed chillies, curry powder, turmeric and salt to the saucepan and cook for a further 5 minutes.

5. Add the finely chopped tomatoes, the eggplant and the water and cook, stirring occasionally, until the vegetables are tender.

6. Stir in the cooked channa dahl and the chopped kale and stir until cooked through, adding a little more water if necessary.

7. Add the coconut milk powder and combine well.

8. Remove from heat, add the coriander (cilantro) and serve.

SERVING SUGGESTION

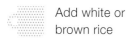 Add white or brown rice

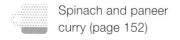 Spinach and paneer curry (page 152)

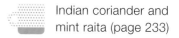 Indian coriander and mint raita (page 233)

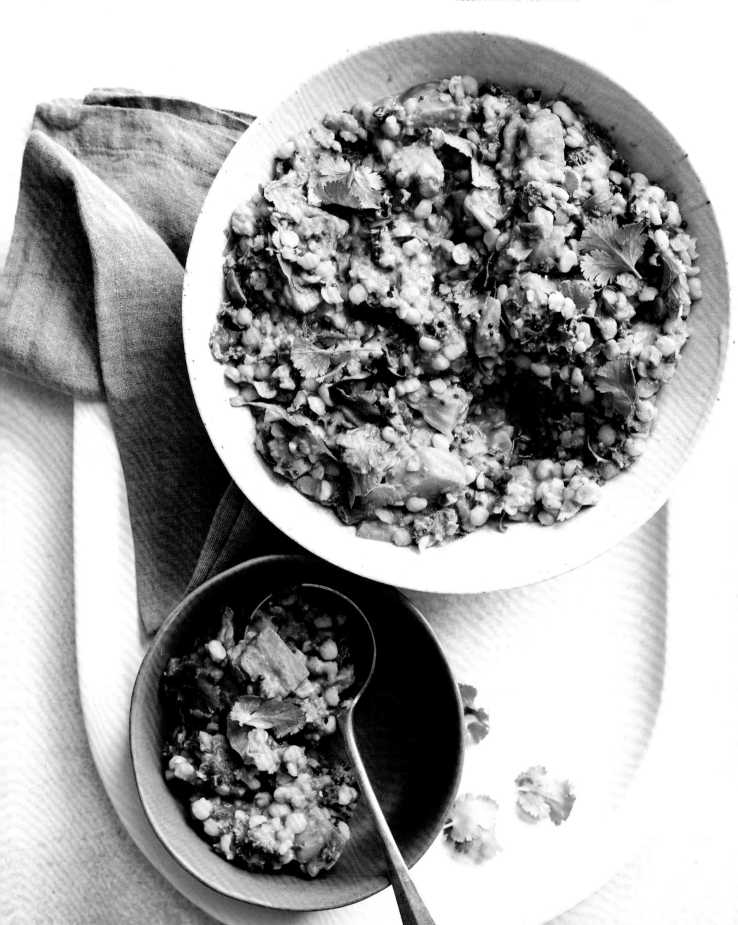

VEGGIE BURGERS

SERVES 6

400g (14oz) peeled sweet potato,
   cut into 3cm (1¼ inch) chunks
180g (6oz) halloumi, grated
1 medium-sized carrot, grated
1 tsp cumin
2 tbsp parsley, roughly chopped
2 tbsp mint leaves, roughly chopped
2 tbsp gluten-free flour
2 tbsp olive oil
lemon wedges and mint leaves
   to garnish

DRESSING

½ cup lactose-free plain yoghurt
1 tsp garlic-infused olive oil
2 tbsp tahini
1 tbsp lemon juice
½ tsp maple syrup

Energy 1287kJ/308 Calories, Protein
10.1g, Total Fat 21.5g, Saturated Fat 6.1g,
Carbohydrate 21.5g, Sugars 7.8g, Dietary
fibre 3.6g, Calcium 270.0mg, Iron 0.9mg.

1. Place the sweet potato in a large saucepan and cover with water. Bring to the boil and cook for 10–15 minutes or until tender. Drain and run the potatoes under cold water to cool.

2. Return the sweet potato to the saucepan.

3. Place the halloumi, mashed sweet potato, carrot, cumin, parsley and mint in a medium-sized bowl and stir to combine. Mix in the gluten-free flour until well combined. Using your hands, form 6 patties and set aside.

4. To make the tahini dressing, combine all of the ingredients in a small bowl and set aside.

5. Heat the olive oil in a large non-stick frypan over medium heat. Fry the patties for 5 minutes on each side or until golden brown.

6. Serve the patties with tahini dressing garnished with lemon wedges and mint leaves.

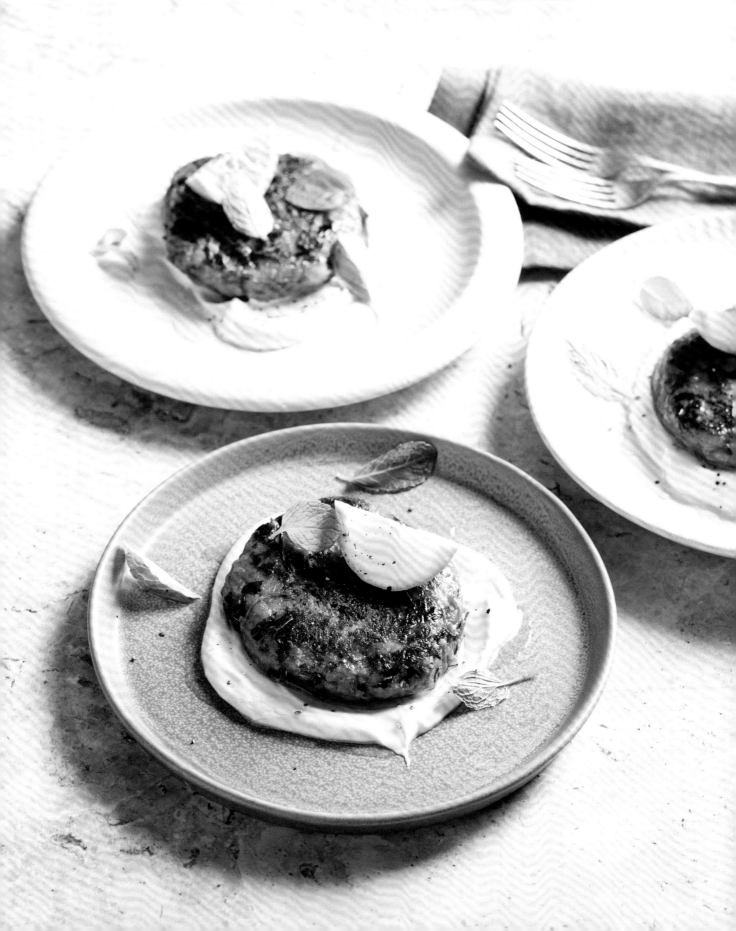

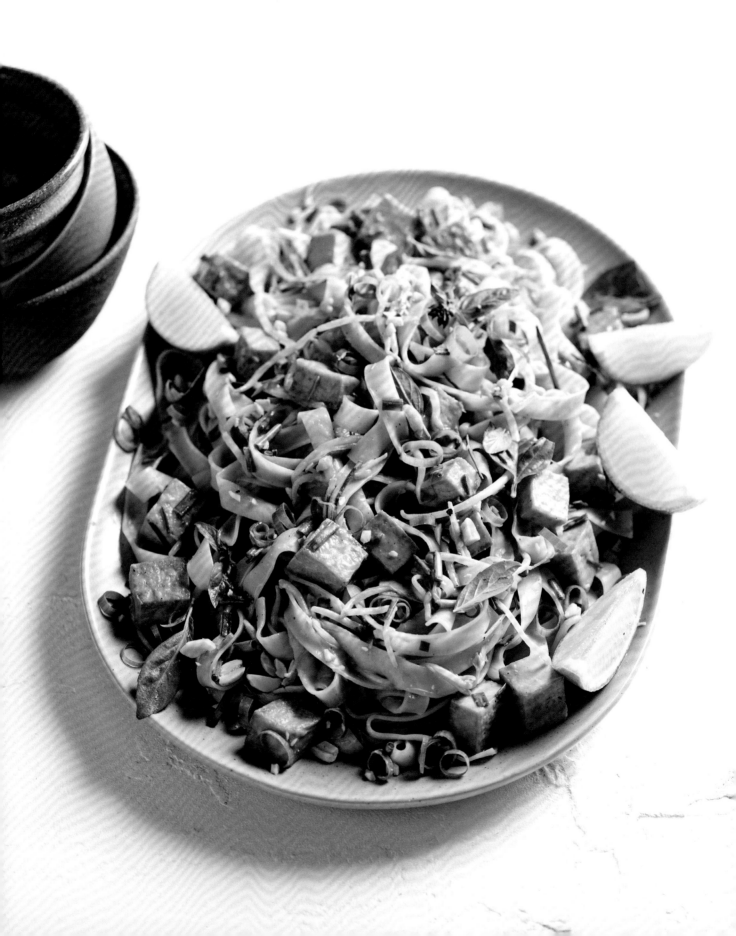

PAD THAI

SERVES 4

250g (9oz) rice noodles
2 tbsp garlic-infused olive oil
200g (7oz) firm tofu, cubed
2 tbsp peanut butter
2 tbsp Asian garlic chives
⅓ cup soy sauce
2 tbsp maple syrup
2 tbsp lime juice
½ cup water
2 cups bean sprouts
¼ cup spring onions (scallions) (green tops only), finely chopped
2 tbsp crushed peanuts to serve
lime wedges to serve

Energy 1734kJ/414 Calories, Protein 14.4g, Total Fat 22.7g, Saturated Fat 3.2g, Carbohydrate 22.7g, Sugars 10.1g, Dietary fibre 5.4g, Calcium 214.0mg, Iron 3.2mg.

1. Add the noodles to a pot of boiling water. Cook for 4–5 minutes or until the noodles are almost tender but still firm. Drain and set aside.

2. Heat the oil in a frypan over medium-high heat. Add the tofu and cook for 2–3 minutes on each side or until lightly browned.

3. Move the tofu to the side of the pan, reduce the heat to medium and add the noodles, peanut butter, garlic chives, soy sauce, maple syrup and lime juice.

4. Stir the noodles until the sauce has thickened slightly and the noodles have cooked through, gradually adding the water if needed, a tablespoon at a time, to stop the noodles from sticking to the pan.

5. Stir in the tofu, bean sprouts and spring onion (scallion) tops.

6. Serve with crushed peanuts and lime wedges.

SAN CHOY BAU

SERVES 4

100g (3½oz) quinoa
1 tbsp garlic-infused olive oil
1 tsp sesame oil
1 tbsp finely grated ginger
1 long red chilli, diced
500g (1lb) firm tofu, crumbled
½ cup Shaoxing wine
¼ cup low FODMAP vegetable
   stock or water
¼ cup kecap manis
220g (8oz) water chestnuts,
   thinly sliced
12 lettuce leaves (butter, cos
   or iceberg)
1 carrot, shredded
1 cup bean sprouts
¼ cup coriander (cilantro)

Energy 1286kJ/307 Calories, Protein 13g,
Total Fat 12.8g, Saturated Fat 2.0g,
Carbohydrate 29.5g, Sugars 19.0 g, Dietary
fibre 9.0g, Calcium 278.0mg, Iron 5.2mg.

1. Cook the quinoa according to packet instructions and set aside.

2. Heat the garlic-infused olive oil in a wok over high heat, add the sesame oil, ginger and chilli and stir-fry for 2–3 minutes.

3. Add the tofu to the wok and stir-fry for 3–5 minutes or until golden. Add the wine, stock or water and kecap manis and cook for 2–3 minutes or until the liquid has slightly reduced. Stir in the quinoa and water chestnuts.

4. To serve, divide the tofu mixture between the lettuce cups. Garnish with carrot, bean sprouts and coriander (cilantro).

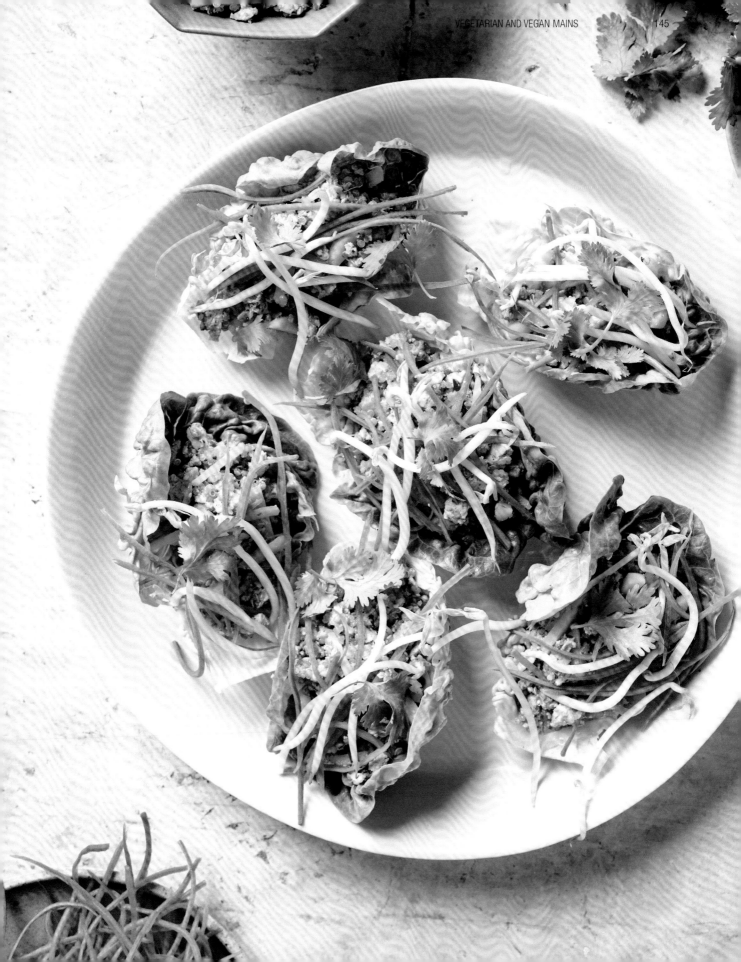

SWEET POTATO OKONOMIYAKI

SERVES 3

1 cup gluten-free flour

½ tsp baking powder

pinch of salt

3 eggs

¾ cup low FODMAP vegetable stock

1 tbsp soy sauce

3 cups shredded wombok (Chinese
   cabbage)

150g (5oz) peeled sweet potato
   peeled and grated

3 tbsp vegetable oil

Japanese tonkatsu sauce to serve
   (see 'basics' page 237)

Japanese mayonnaise to serve

¼ cup spring onions (scallions)
   (green tops only), finely sliced

1 tsp toasted sesame seeds to serve

Energy 2039kJ/487 Calories, Protein
11.0g, Total Fat 26.0g, Saturated Fat 3.7g,
Carbohydrate 50.8g, Sugars 10.1g, Dietary
fibre 2.9g, Calcium 75.1mg, Iron 2.3mg.

1. In a large bowl, whisk together the flour, baking powder and
    pinch of salt. Add the eggs, stock, and soy sauce and beat
    until combined.

2. Stir in the cabbage, sweet potato and spring onion
    (scallion) tops.

3. In a large non-stick frypan, heat 1 tbsp of the oil over medium
    heat. Using a spatula, ladle a third of the batter into
    the pan to form a pancake.

4. Cook the pancake for 3–4 minutes on each side or until golden
    brown, turning once. Transfer the pancake to a plate lined with
    paper towel.

5. Repeat with the remaining oil and batter to make two
    more pancakes.

6. To serve, drizzle the pancakes with tonkatsu sauce and mayo,
    scatter with sesame seeds and top with finely sliced spring
    onion tops.

SERVING SUGGESTION

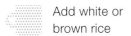 Add white or
brown rice

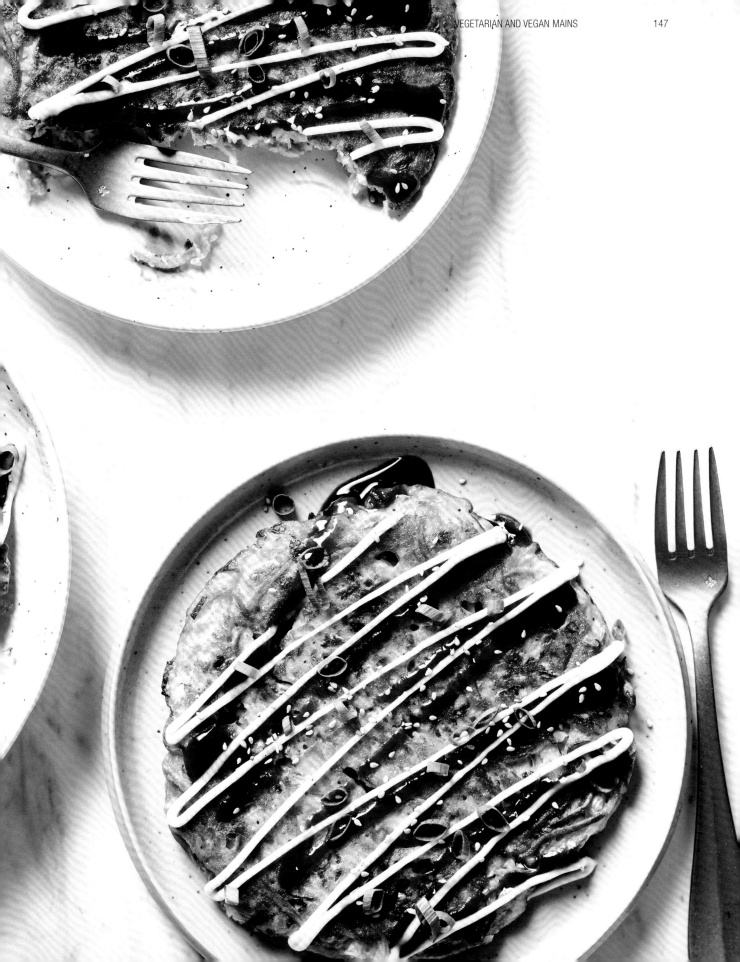

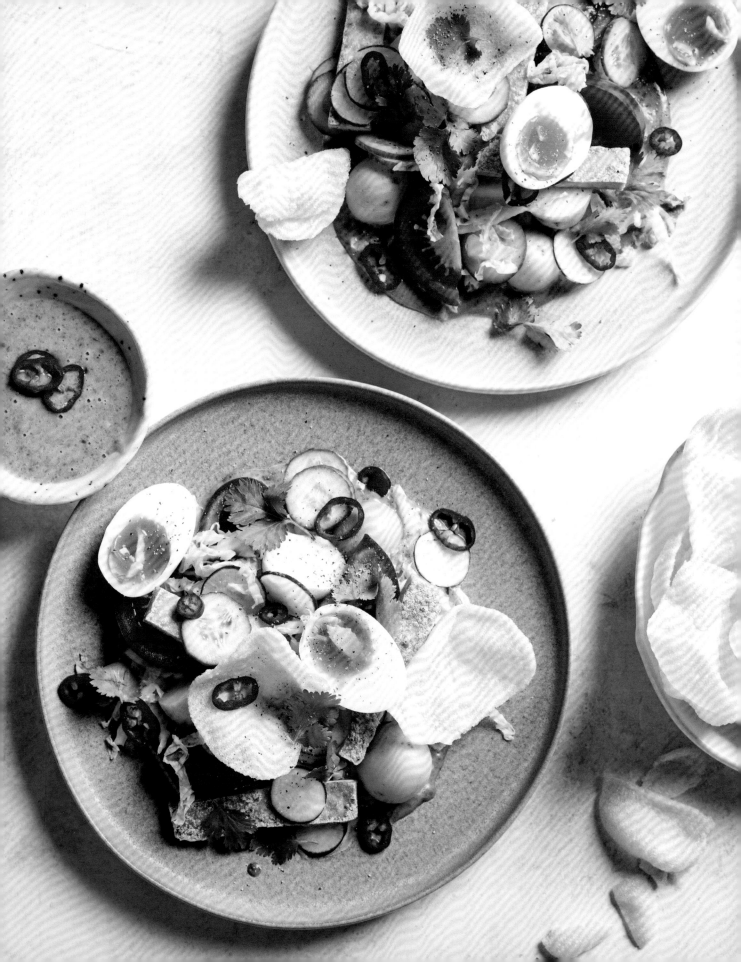

GADO GADO

SERVES 4

SALAD
400g (14oz) baby or 'new' potatoes
4 large eggs
400g (14oz) firm tofu, cut into 2½cm
    (1 inch) dice
1 tbsp sesame oil
salt and pepper to taste
half a wombok (Chinese cabbage),
    shredded
2 fresh tomatoes (common/truss),
    sliced into wedges
4 radishes, thinly sliced
1 Lebanese cucumber, thinly sliced
½ cup coriander (cilantro)
1 large chilli, finely sliced
12 prawn crackers (optional) (without
    garlic or onion)

SAUCE
50g (2oz) palm sugar, grated
½ cup crunchy peanut butter
1 large red chilli, finely sliced

Energy 1515kJ/362 Calories, Protein
23.5g, Total Fat 18.1g, Saturated Fat 5.7g,
Carbohydrate 23.1g, Sugars 5.7g, Dietary
fibre 8.3g, Calcium 421.3mg, Iron 6.1mg.

1. Cook the potatoes in boiling water for approximately 15 minutes or until cooked through. Slice the potatoes in half.

2. Boil the eggs to your liking (approximately 7 minutes for soft-boiled and 9 minutes for hard-boiled). Peel, halve and set aside.

3. Heat the sesame oil in a frypan over medium heat. Add the tofu and cook, turning occasionally, for 5–10 minutes, or until browned all over. Season with salt and pepper and set aside.

4. Place the cabbage in a large colander and slowly pour a kettle of boiling water over it to cook the cabbage slightly. Transfer the cabbage to a large bowl.

5. Add the tomato, radishes and cucumber and season to taste with salt and pepper. Set aside.

6. To make the sauce, place the palm sugar, peanut butter and chilli into a food processor and blitz until smooth.

7. Divide the sauce mixture between four serving bowls and arrange the salad ingredients, tofu and eggs over the top.

8. To serve, garnish with coriander leaves and finely sliced fresh chilli. Top with prawn crackers (optional).

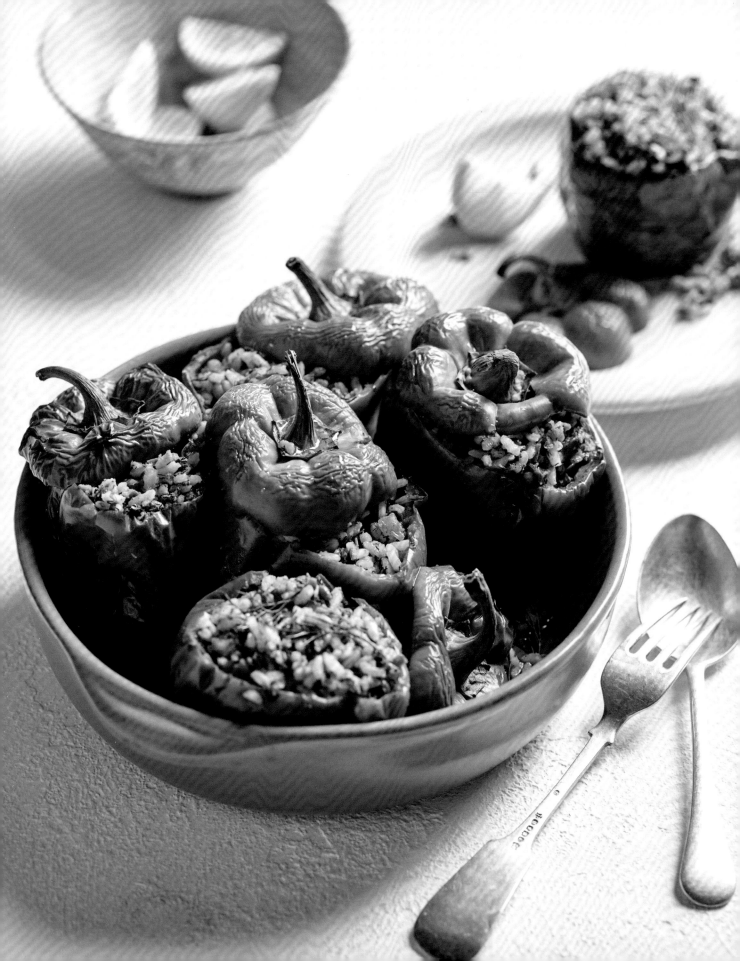

STUFFED CAPSICUMS

SERVES 6

¼ cup pine nuts, toasted

6 medium-sized green capsicums (bell peppers)

1 cup medium grain white rice

2 tbsp garlic-infused olive oil

1 cup canned lentils, drained and rinsed

2 medium tomatoes (common/truss), finely chopped

1 tsp cumin

1 tsp allspice

1 tsp sweet paprika

¼ tsp pepper

1 cup parsley, roughly chopped

½ cup dill

lemon wedges to serve

Energy 1568kJ/375 Calories, Protein 12.1g, Total Fat 15.4g, Saturated Fat 1.6g, Carbohydrate 42.1g, Sugars 8.2g, Dietary fibre 9.1g, Calcium 56.2mg, Iron 3.4mg.

1. Preheat the oven to 200°C/400°F.

2. Cut the tops from the capsicums (bell peppers) and reserve. Remove the seeds and white membrane and discard. Cook the capsicums and their lids in a pot of boiling salted water for 10–15 minutes or until softened. Drain and set aside.

3. Cook the rice according to packet instructions, then set aside to cool slightly. Heat the garlic-infused olive oil in a large saucepan over medium heat. Add the lentils, tomato, spices, herbs and pine nuts and stir for 3–4 minutes or until fragrant. Stir in the rice.

4. Stuff each capsicum with filling, cover with the tops and place in an ovenproof dish. Bake for 20–25 minutes or until light golden.

SERVING SUGGESTION

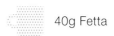 40g Fetta

SPINACH AND PANEER CURRY

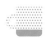

SERVES 6

1 tsp turmeric

½ tsp cayenne pepper

salt to taste

4½ tbsp garlic-infused olive oil

240g (8½oz) paneer cheese, cut into
2cm (¾ inch) cubes

250g (9oz) frozen spinach, thawed

½ cup spring onions (scallions) (green
tops only), finely chopped

1 tbsp finely grated ginger

1 green chilli, finely chopped

½ tsp garam masala

2 tsp ground coriander

1 tsp cumin

½ cup lactose-free Greek yoghurt

1 tbsp coriander (cilantro) leaves
to garnish

Energy 1262kJ/302 Calories, Protein
10.2g, Total Fat 25.6g, Saturated Fat 9.9g,
Carbohydrate 7.6g, Sugars 2.5g, Dietary
fibre 2.5g, Calcium 245.0mg, Iron 3.8mg.

1. To make the spice mixture, combine the turmeric,
cayenne pepper, salt and 3 tbsp of garlic-infused olive oil
in a small bowl.

2. Add the paneer cheese to the spice mixture, a few cubes at
a time, and stir gently with a spoon or with your hands to coat
the cheese in spices. Transfer the cubes to another bowl as
you go, and set aside to marinate.

3. Blitz the thawed spinach in a food processor until smooth.
Set aside.

4. Heat a large heavy-based non-stick pan over medium
heat. Add the paneer and spice mixture and cook, turning
occasionally, until the paneer is browned on all sides.
Remove from pan and set aside.

5. Return the pan to the heat and reduce the heat to low. Add the
remaining 1½ tbsp oil, spring onion tops, ginger and chopped
green chilli. Cook gently over low heat for 10–15 minutes, or
until the spring onion tops are wilted and the mixture is fragrant,
stirring occasionally. Add water if necessary to stop the mixture
from sticking.

6. Add the garam masala, coriander and cumin and stir for 5
minutes or until fragrant.

7. Add the pureed spinach and the ½ cup water and cook for 5
minutes or until heated through.

8. Remove the pan from the heat and stir through the yoghurt.
Add the cooked paneer cubes and stir gently to combine.
Serve scattered with coriander leaves.

SERVING SUGGESTION

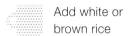 Add white or
brown rice

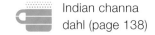 Indian channa
dahl (page 138)

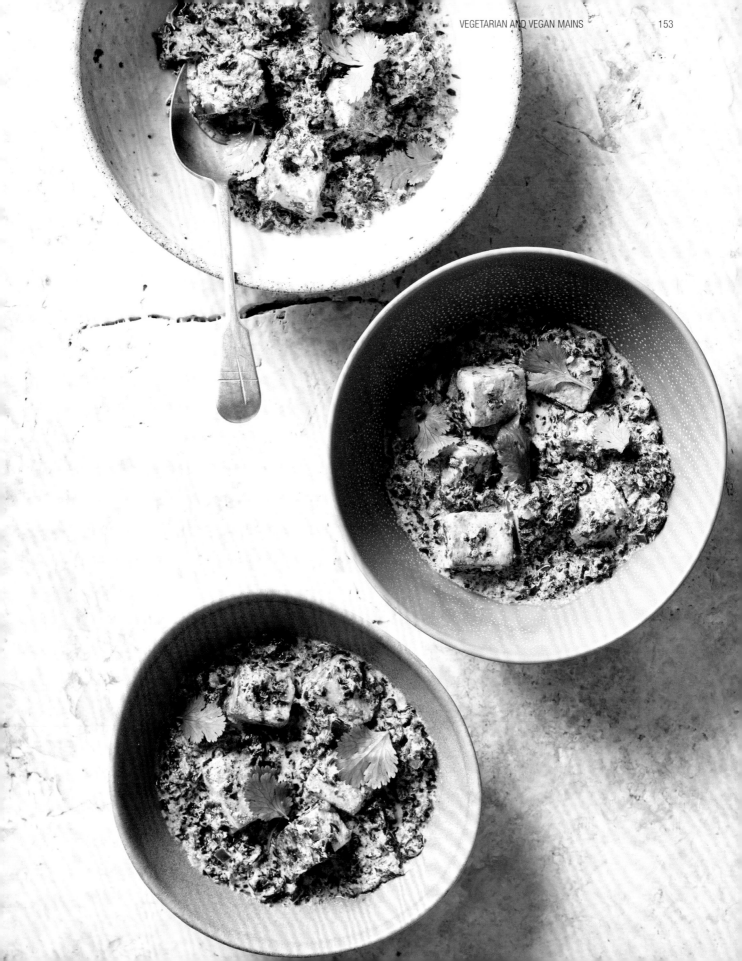

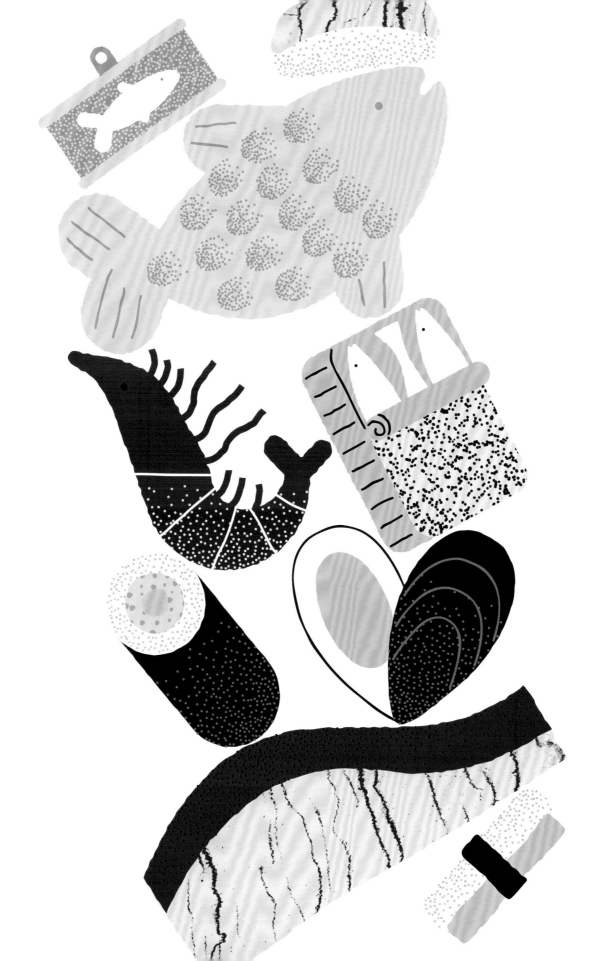

FISH

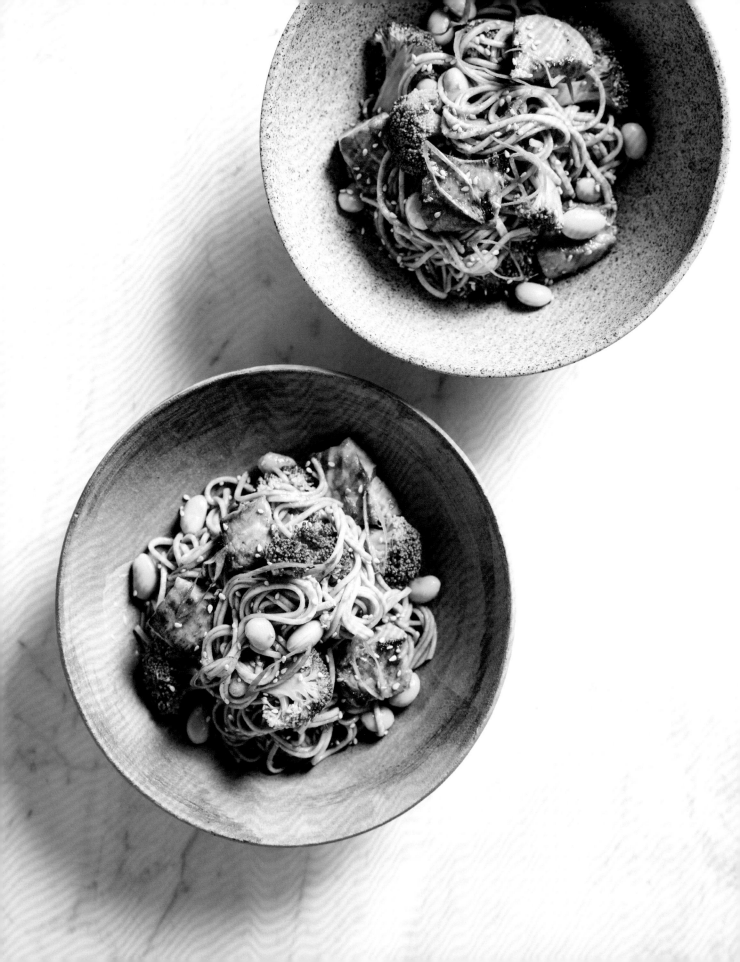

SALMON AND SOBA NOODLE STIR-FRY

SERVES 4

1 tbsp grated ginger

1 tbsp sesame oil

1 tbsp mirin

¼ cup soy sauce

600g (1lb 3oz) salmon fillet, skin removed, cubed

300g (10½oz) soba noodles

1 tbsp peanut oil

¼ cup Chinese rice wine

300g (10½oz) broccoli, heads only

200g (7oz) frozen edamame

¼ cup water

¼ cup spring onions (scallions) (green tops only), finely sliced

1 tbsp sesame seeds

Energy 3453kJ/825 Calories, Protein 49.1g, Total Fat 44.9g, Saturated Fat 8.8g, Carbohydrate 51.1g, Sugars 5.1g, Dietary fibre 8.2g, Calcium 147.3mg, Iron 3.9mg.

1. Combine the ginger, sesame oil, mirin and 2 tbsp soy sauce in a bowl. Toss the salmon in the marinade and set aside for approximately 20 minutes.

2. Meanwhile, cook the soba noodles according to packet instructions.

3. Heat ½ tbsp of the peanut oil in a wok over high heat. Add half of the salmon and stir-fry for 2-3 minutes or until cooked through. Repeat the process with the remaining salmon and oil. Cover with foil and set aside.

4. Add the rice wine, broccoli, edamame, remaining soy sauce and ¼ cup water to the wok. Stir for 3–4 minutes or until the liquid has partially reduced.

5. Add the noodles and salmon, including any juices. Remove from the heat and stir to combine.

6. Serve topped with spring onion (scallion) tops and sesame seeds.

MIDDLE EASTERN FISH WITH TAHINI SAUCE

  (GF) (Pr) (Ca) (Fe) (DF)

SERVES 5

1kg (2lb) firm white fish fillets (such
    as snapper or blue-eye trevalla)
¼ cup pine nuts

CORIANDER PASTE

30g (1oz) coriander (cilantro)
½ cup spring onions (scallions)
    (green tops only)
1 tsp chilli flakes
¼ cup lemon juice
¼ cup garlic-infused olive oil

TAHINI SAUCE

150g (5oz) tahini
1 tbsp ground coriander
1 tsp chilli powder
¼ cup water
½ cup lemon juice
1 tbsp garlic-infused olive oil
salt and pepper to taste
¼ cup parsley, roughly chopped,
    to serve

1. Preheat the oven to 200°C/400°F.

2. To make the coriander paste, place the coriander (cilantro), spring onion (scallion) tops, chilli flakes, lemon juice and garlic-infused olive oil into a food processor. Pulse until a paste forms.

3. Rub the paste evenly over each fish fillet and place on a baking tray. Cover with foil and place in the oven. Bake for 25 minutes or until the fish is cooked through.

4. While the fish is cooking, toast the pine nuts in a small pan for 1-2 minutes or until golden brown.

5. To make the tahini sauce, place the tahini, ground coriander, chilli powder, lemon juice, water, salt and pepper in a saucepan over medium heat and bring to the boil.

6. Reduce the heat to low and simmer the sauce for 10 minutes or until it has thickened slightly. Add more water if needed for a sauce consistency.

7. Divide the fish between serving plates and pour over the tahini sauce. Serve topped with pine nuts and parsley.

Energy 2322kJ/555 Calories, Protein 46.8g, Total Fat 37.5g, Saturated Fat 5.1g, Carbohydrate 4.6g, Sugars 4.1g, Dietary fibre 6.6g, Calcium 201.0mg, Iron 3.6mg.

SERVING SUGGESTION

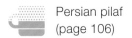 Persian pilaf
(page 106)

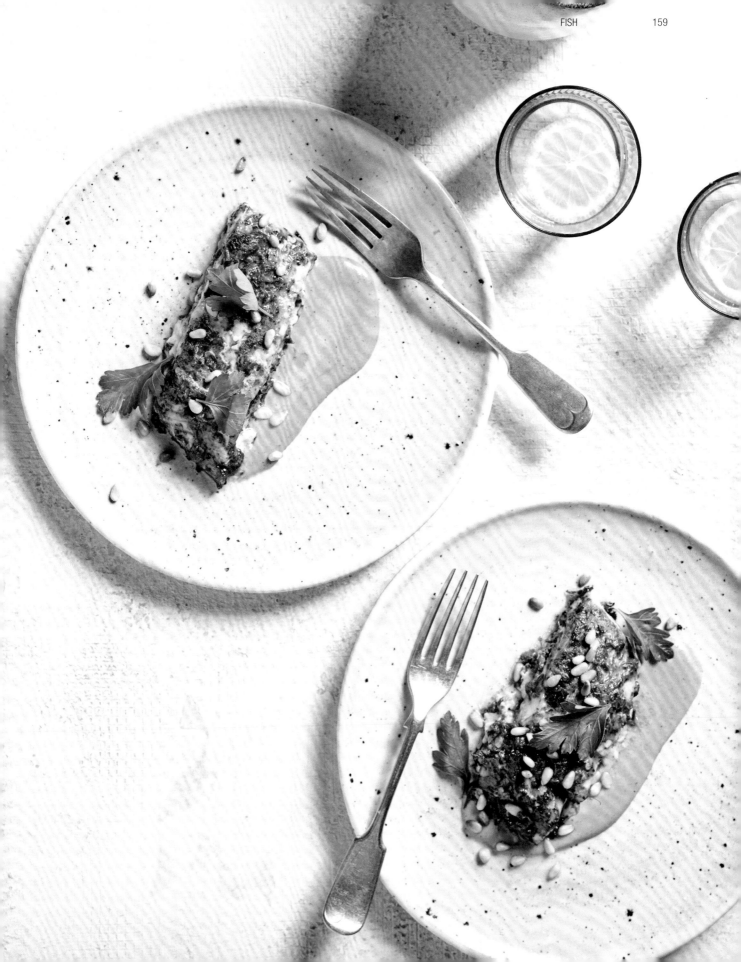

PRAWN WONTONS WITH SICHUAN CHILLI OIL

SERVES 4

20–25 wonton wrappers
water for sealing wrappers

FILLING

300g (10½oz) green prawns, peeled
and deveined
¼ cup spring onions (scallions) (green
tops only), finely chopped
1 tbsp coriander (cilantro),
finely chopped
1 tbsp sesame oil
2 tbsp finely grated ginger

RED OIL SAUCE

¼ cup soy sauce
2 tbsp Chinese black vinegar
2 tbsp Sichuan chilli oil (see 'basics',
page 236)
½ tsp sugar
sesame seeds to serve

Energy 1318kJ/315 Calories, Protein
21.4g, Total Fat 8.9g, Saturated Fat 1.1g,
Carbohydrate 36.1g, Sugars 4.0g, Dietary
fibre 0.5g, Calcium 98.5mg, Iron 0.7mg.

1. To make the filling, finely chop the prawns or mince them in a food processor. Set aside.

2. To make the red oil sauce, combine all the ingredients in a small bowl. Set aside.

3. In a bowl, combine the minced prawns with the spring onion (scallion) tops, coriander (cilantro), sesame oil and ginger.

4. Working with one wonton wrapper at a time, place approximately 1 tsp of the filling in the centre of a wrapper. Brush the edges with water, fold to form a triangle and enclose the filling, and press the edges to seal and remove air. Bring two corners of the triangle together to form a wonton shape and seal with water. Place the wonton on a tray lined with baking paper.

5. Repeat with the remaining wonton wrappers and filling.

6. Cook the wontons in batches in a large saucepan of boiling water for 5 minutes or until they float to the top. Remove the wontons with a slotted spoon and set them aside while you cook the remaining wontons.

7. Pour the sauce over the wontons and toss lightly to coat evenly. Transfer to a serving plate, sprinkle with sesame seeds and serve.

SERVING SUGGESTION

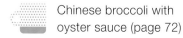 Chinese broccoli with oyster sauce (page 72)

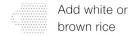 Add white or brown rice

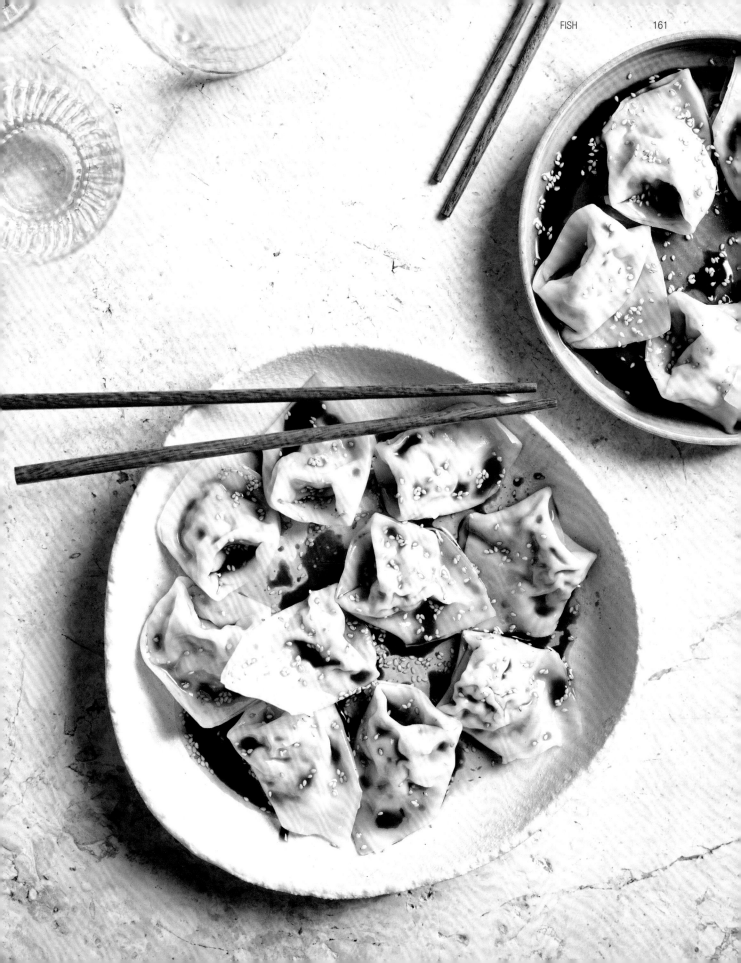

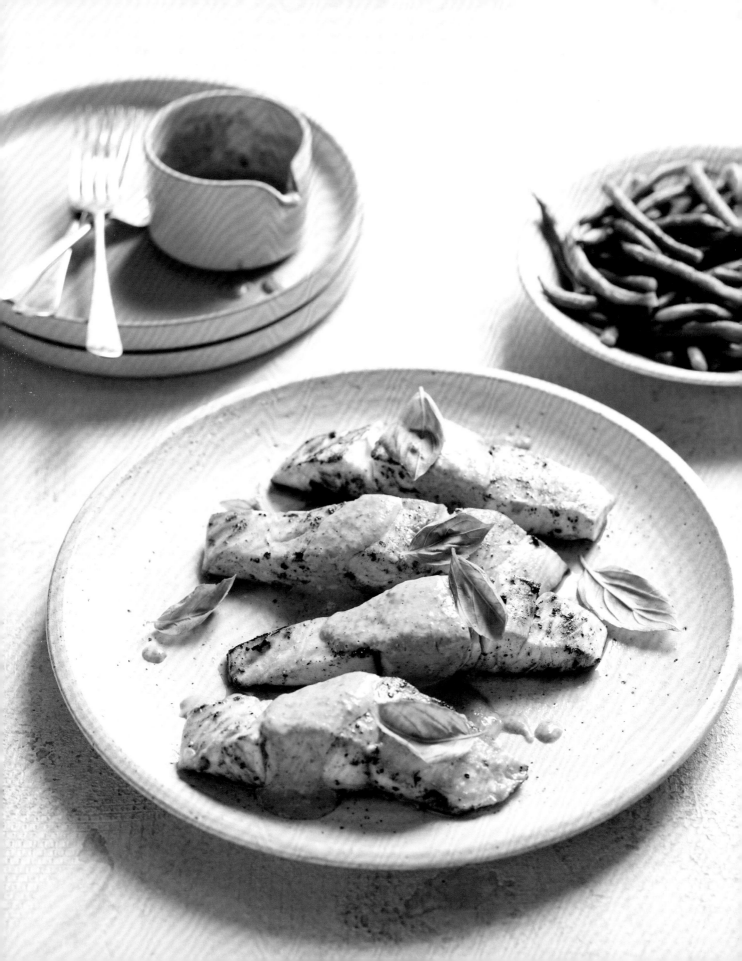

FISH WITH LEMON, BASIL AND GREEN BEANS

SERVES 4
650g (1lb 4oz) centre-cut blue-eye
    trevalla fillets, skin removed
1 lemon, juiced
100ml (3½fl oz) dry white wine
1 cup low FODMAP vegetable stock
1 cup basil leaves
⅓ cup pine nuts, toasted
⅓ cup olive oil
salt and pepper to taste
400g (14oz) green beans, trimmed
¼ cup basil leaves, extra, to garnish

Energy 1858kJ/444 Calories, Protein
36.3g, Total Fat 29.9g, Saturated Fat 4.0g,
Carbohydrate 4.4g, Sugars 3.3g, Dietary
fibre 4.5g, Calcium 112.2mg, Iron 2.7mg.

1. In a shallow dish, toss the fish with the white wine and half the lemon juice. Cover the fish and refrigerate for 20 minutes.

2. Drain the fish well and reserve the marinade juices. Cover the fish and set aside in the fridge. Add the reserved marinade to a saucepan with the stock. Bring to the boil. Reduce heat to medium and cook for 10 minutes or until the liquid has reduced by half. Set aside to cool.

3. Blitz the basil and pine nuts with 2 tbsp of oil in a food processor until smooth. Gradually add the stock mixture and pulse until smooth. Season with salt and pepper. Set the sauce aside and keep warm.

4. Cook the beans in a saucepan of boiling water for approximately 6 minutes or until just tender. Drain, season with salt and pepper and drizzle with remaining lemon juice. Set the beans aside.

5. Heat the remaining 2 tbsp of oil in a large heavy-based pan over medium heat. Season the fish with salt and pepper and cook, turning once, for approximately 8 minutes or until just cooked through.

6. Serve the fish with beans, parsley and basil sauce.

SERVING SUGGESTION

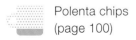
Polenta chips
(page 100)

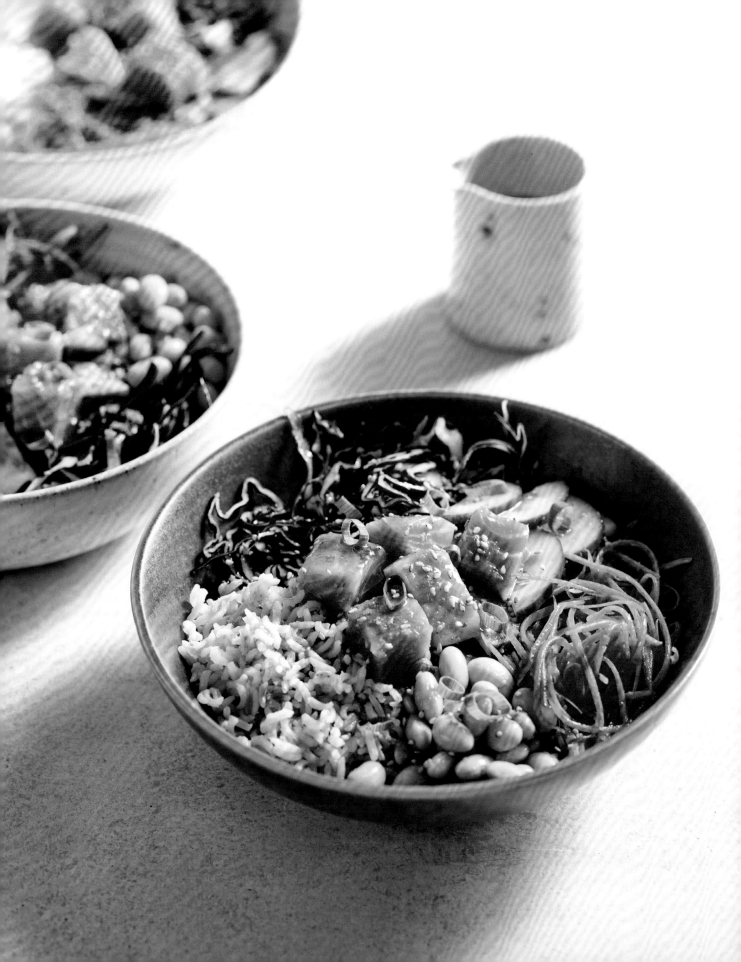

SALMON POKE BOWL

SERVES 4

400g (14oz) sashimi-grade salmon,
  cut into 2cm (¾ inch) cubes
¼ cup spring onions (scallions) (green
  tops only), roughly chopped
4 cups cooked brown rice
200g (7oz) edamame, cooked
  until tender
150g (5oz) red cabbage, shredded
half a cucumber, finely sliced
1 large carrot, grated
1 tbsp sesame seeds to serve

SAUCE

¼ cup soy sauce
2 tbsp rice wine vinegar
½ tbsp sriracha
1 tbsp maple syrup
2 tbsp sesame oil
2 tsp finely grated ginger

Energy 2822kJ/674 Calories, Protein
35.8g, Total Fat 22.3g, Saturated Fat 5.0g,
Carbohydrate 78.4g, Sugars 8.5g, Dietary
fibre 6.0g, Calcium 81.9mg, Iron 2.9mg.

1. Add all sauce ingredients to a small bowl and whisk
    to combine.

2. Combine the salmon, the spring onion (scallion) tops and
    half the sauce in a bowl and gently toss to coat.

3. Divide the rice among four bowls, top with the salmon,
    edamame, red cabbage, cucumber and carrot. Sprinkle over
    the sesame seeds and serve with the remaining sauce on
    the side.

SERVING SUGGESTION

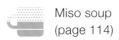
Miso soup
(page 114)

LEMON AND PARSLEY STEAMED MUSSELS

SERVES 2

1kg (2lb) large mussels, uncooked

1 tbsp garlic-infused olive oil

3 tsp butter

1 cup spring onions (scallions) (green tops only), finely chopped

1 cup dry white wine

1 tbsp lemon juice

¼ cup parsley, finely chopped

lemon wedges to serve

salt and ground black pepper to taste

Energy 1884kJ/450 Calories, Protein 32.1g, Total Fat 20.8g, Saturated Fat 5.1g, Carbohydrate 11.6g, Sugars 2.5g, Dietary fibre 0.9g, Calcium 295.1mg, Iron 7.6mg.

1. Wash the mussels in cold water. Remove the mussel 'beards' and set aside.

2. Preheat a heavy-based casserole dish with a well-fitting lid over low heat. Add the oil, butter and spring onion (scallion) tops and sauté for 2–3 minutes or until softened.

3. Increase the heat to high, add the white wine and bring to the boil. Pour in the washed mussels and cover with the lid. Cook for 5 minutes or until the mussels have opened. Using tongs, transfer the opened mussels to a serving platter. Discard any unopened mussels.

4. Strain the juices from the casserole dish through a fine sieve and pour them over the mussels along with the lemon juice. Serve the mussels with parsley, lemon wedges, and salt and pepper to taste.

SERVING SUGGESTION

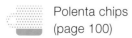
Polenta chips
(page 100)

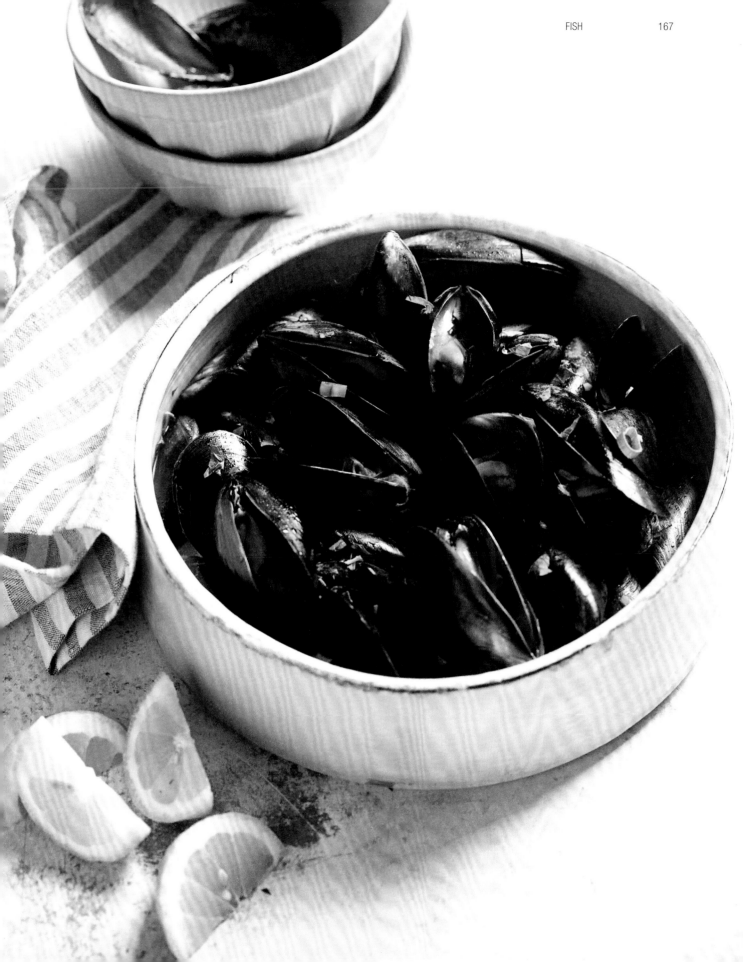

BAKED FISH WITH GINGER SESAME AND SOY

SERVES 4

4 firm white fish fillets (such as
   snapper, bass, hapuku, rockling)
   (approximately 800g/1lb 12oz total)
2 tbsp Shaoxing wine
1 tbsp sesame oil
salt and pepper to taste
5cm (2 inches) ginger, peeled
   and julienned
¼ cup spring onions (scallions)
   (green tops only)
¼ cup coriander
1 long red chilli, julienned

SAUCE

1½ tbsp sesame oil
¼ cup soy sauce
½ tsp sugar
1 tbsp Shaoxing wine

Energy 1527kJ/365 Calories, Protein
48.2g, Total Fat 17.7g, Saturated Fat 3.3g,
Carbohydrate 2.1g, Sugars 1.3g, Dietary
fibre 1.1g, Calcium 99.3mg, Iron 1.6mg.

1. Preheat the oven to 200°C/400°F.

2. Place each fish fillet on a piece of baking paper large enough
    to wrap the fish. Drizzle the sesame oil and Shaoxing wine over
    the fish. Season with salt and pepper.

3. Scatter the julienned ginger over the fish.

4. Fold the paper to wrap each fish fillet, taking care to enclose
    it completely.

5. Place the fish on a baking tray and bake for 10–15 minutes or
    until the fish is cooked through and opaque. If the fish is still
    translucent, cook for an additional
    2–3 minutes.

6. While the fish is cooking, prepare the sauce by combining the
    sesame oil, soy sauce, sugar and Shaoxing wine in a bowl.

7. Take the fish out of the oven and open each parcel. Pour the
    sauce over the fish.

8. Serve garnished with fresh coriander (cilantro), spring onion
    (scallion) tops and julienned red chilli.

SERVING SUGGESTION

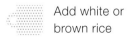 Add white or
brown rice

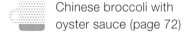 Chinese broccoli with
oyster sauce (page 72)

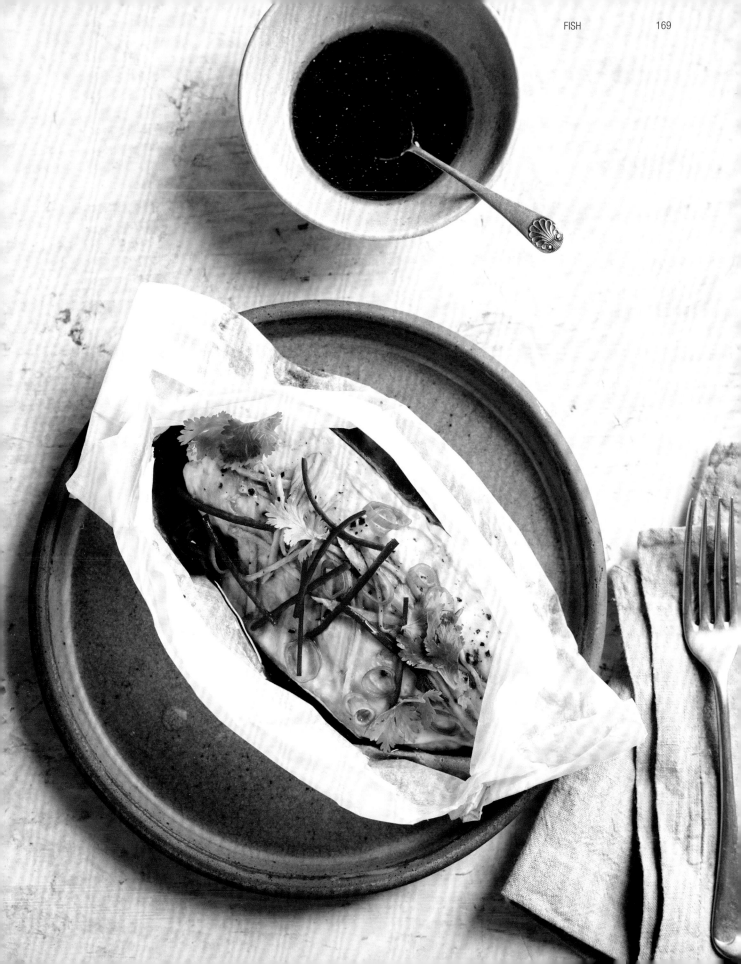

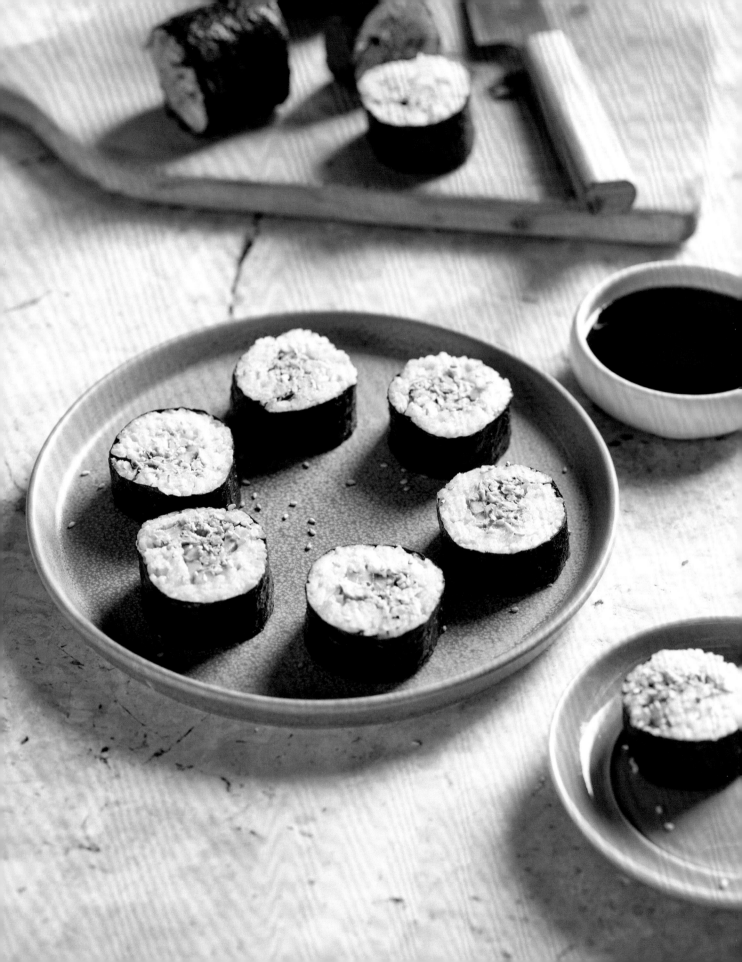

TUNA ROLLS

 (Pr)

SERVES 3

1 cup sushi rice

2½ tbsp rice wine vinegar

2 tsp sugar

1 tsp sea salt

200g (7oz) canned tuna, drained

2 tbsp Japanese mayonnaise

1 tbsp sriracha sauce

2 tsp sesame oil

2 tsp soy sauce

1 tbsp finely chopped chives

3 sheets nori seaweed

¼ cucumber, cut into batons

1 tbsp sesame seeds

¼ cup soy sauce to serve

Energy 2143kJ/512 Calories, Protein
25.9g, Total Fat 17.7g, Saturated Fat 3.1g,
Carbohydrate 60.0g, Sugars 4.9g, Dietary
fibre 2.3g, Calcium 35.6mg, Iron 2.4mg.

1. Cook the rice according to packet instructions. While the rice is cooking, combine the rice wine vinegar, sugar and salt in a small bowl, microwave for 20 seconds and stir until sugar dissolves.

2. Once the rice is cooked, transfer to a wooden or plastic bowl and pour over the vinegar mixture. Stir with a wooden spoon and set rice aside to cool to room temperature.

3. In a bowl, whisk together the Japanese mayonnaise, sriracha, sesame oil, soy sauce and chives. Add the tuna and stir to combine. Set aside.

4. To make the sushi rolls, place a nori seaweed sheet, shiny side down, on a bamboo sushi rolling mat or a piece of baking paper folded in half over a clean tea towel. Press a third of the rice evenly over the sheet, leaving approximately 2cm (¾ inch) of space at the farthest edge.

5. Place 2–3 cucumber sticks in the centre of the rice and spoon a third of the tuna mixture on top.

6. Starting at the edge of the sushi roll closest to you, firmly roll the sushi roll away from you, using the sushi mat or tea towel to help you roll. Press down firmly to seal at the end and set aside. Repeat with the remaining two nori sheets and filling.

7. Place the sushi rolls on a cutting board. Using a very sharp knife dipped in cold water, and rewetting the knife between cuts, cut the rolls in half and in half again.

8. Place the sushi rolls on a serving platter and sprinkle with sesame seeds. Serve with soy sauce for dipping.

THAI FISH CAKES

SERVES 4 (MAKES 12)

500g (1lb) white fish fillets

3 tbsp low FODMAP red curry paste
(see 'basics', page 235)

2 tbsp coriander (cilantro) leaves

1 tbsp fish sauce

1 tbsp lime juice

1 egg

½ cup rice flour

50g (2oz) green beans, finely chopped

3 tbsp vegetable oil

lime wedges to serve

sweet chilli sauce to serve

Energy 1606kJ/384 Calories, Protein
29.3g, Total Fat 21.8g, Saturated Fat 3.1g,
Carbohydrate 16.4g, Sugars 1.3g, Dietary
fibre 2.0g, Calcium 98.9mg, Iron 1.9mg.

1. Add the fish, curry paste, coriander (cilantro), fish sauce, lime juice and egg to a food processor. Blitz until a paste forms.

2. Place the paste into a mixing bowl. Mix through the rice flour and chopped green beans until thoroughly combined.

3. Wet your hands, take a ¼ cup of the mixture at a time and use your hands to form patties 1cm (½ inch) thick.

4. Heat a frypan over medium heat with enough oil to cover the base. Working in batches, add the fish patties to the oil and cook for 3–4 minutes on each side or until golden brown, then transfer to a plate lined with paper towel.

5. Repeat with remaining patties, adding more oil to the pan as necessary.

6. Serve with lime wedges and sweet chilli sauce.

SERVING SUGGESTION

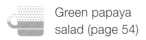
Green papaya
salad (page 54)

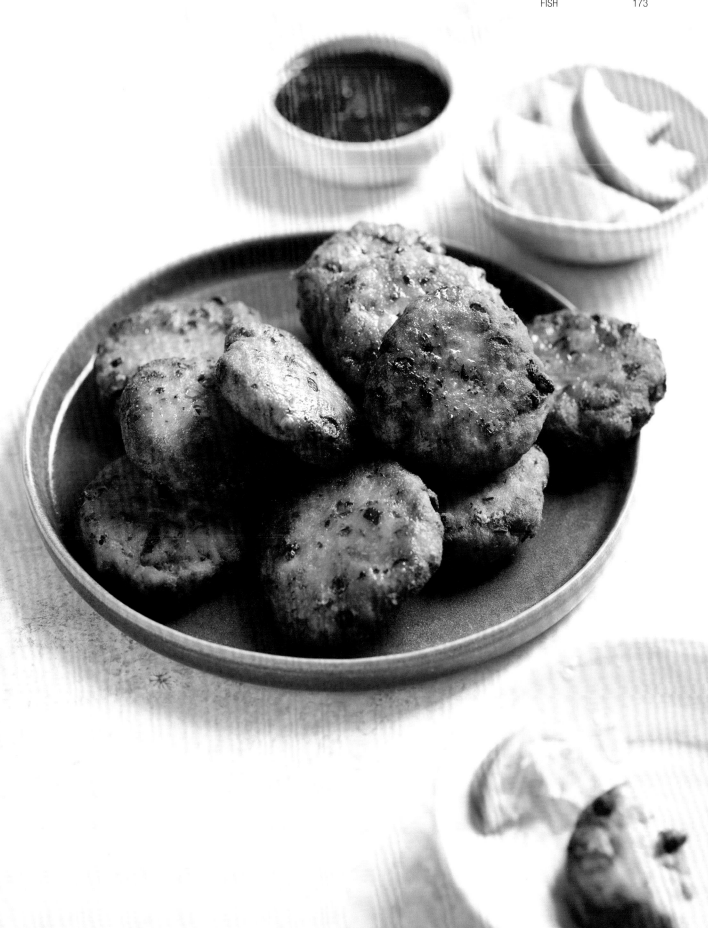
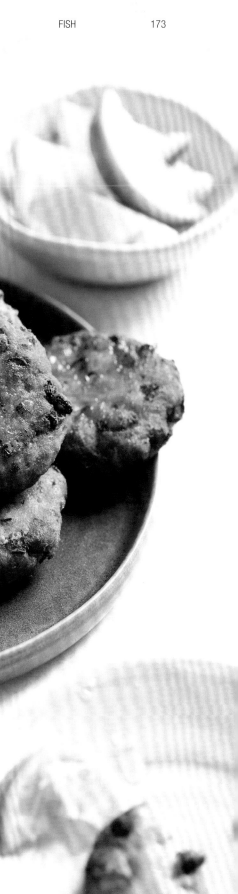

THAI CRISPY FISH

SERVES 5

750g (1lb 7oz) fish fillets (firm
    white fish)
⅓ cup garlic-infused oil

SAUCE

2 cups roughly chopped spring onion
    (scallion) tops
3 tsp finely grated ginger
½ tsp crushed dried chilli
2 tbsp light soy sauce
1 tbsp palm sugar
1 tbsp lemon juice
1 tbsp fish sauce
¼ tsp ground black pepper
½ cup coriander (cilantro) leaves
    to garnish

Energy 1275kJ/305 Calories, Protein
30.5g, Total Fat 18.7g, Saturated Fat 3.3g,
Carbohydrate 3.3g, Sugars 3.0g, Dietary
fibre 1.0g, Calcium 68.4mg, Iron 0.9mg.

1. Heat the oil in a frypan over medium-high heat and fry the fish until lightly browned and crispy on both sides. Transfer the cooked fish to a serving platter and keep warm.

2. To make the sauce, lower the heat and allow the oil to cool slightly before adding the chopped spring onion (scallion) tops, grated ginger and chilli. Fry on low heat until soft. Add the soy sauce, palm sugar, lemon juice, fish sauce and pepper and simmer for 1-2 minutes, stirring to dissolve the sugar.

3. Pour the sauce over the cooked fish and sprinkle with coriander (cilantro) leaves. Serve immediately.

SERVING SUGGESTION

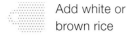 Add white or
brown rice

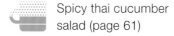 Spicy thai cucumber
salad (page 61)

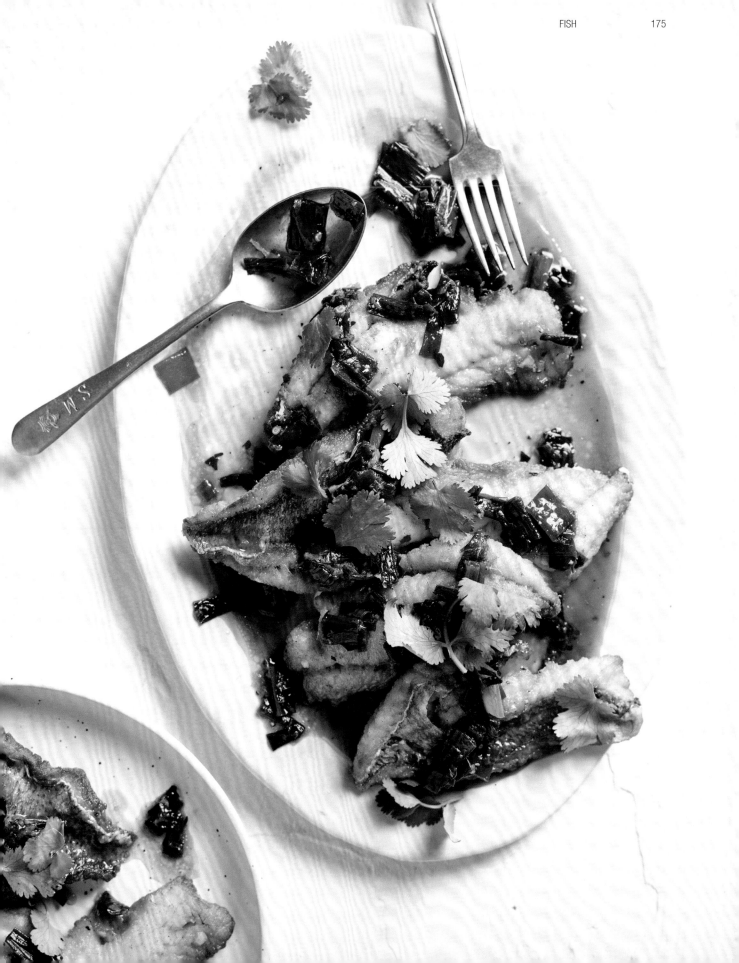

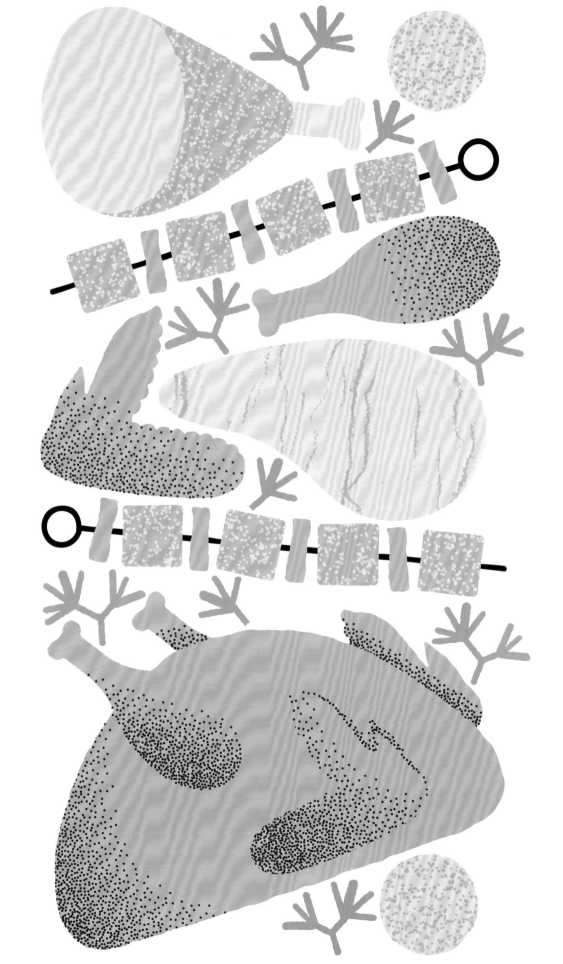

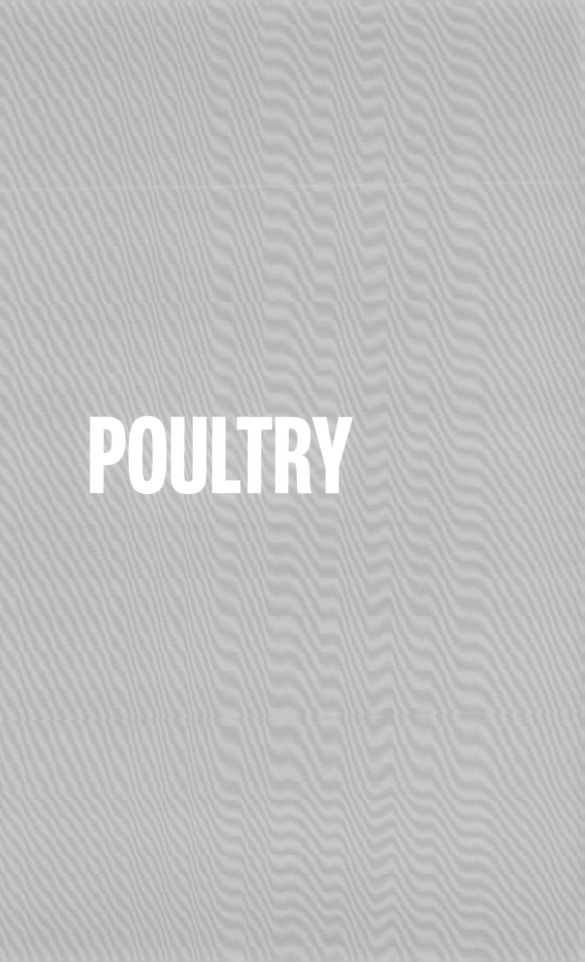

POULTRY

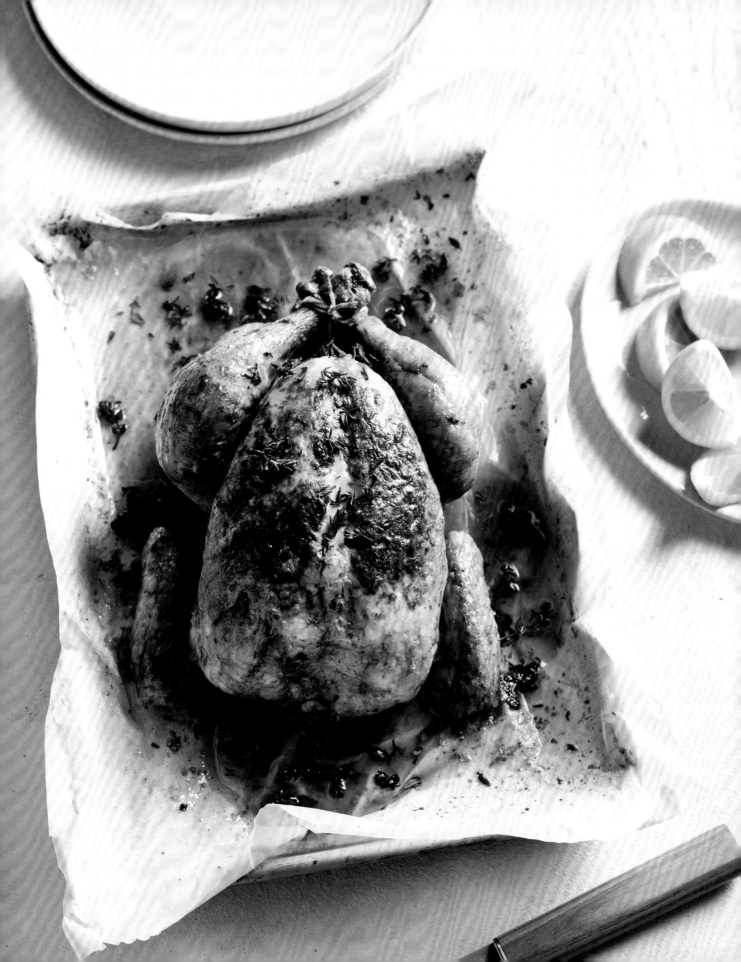

HERBY ROAST CHICKEN

SERVES 4

1 whole chicken (1.5kg/3lb 3oz)
¼ cup parsley leaves, roughly chopped
1 tbsp garlic-infused olive oil
sea salt to taste
1 lemon, halved
½ small bunch thyme
4 rosemary sprigs
2 tbsp extra virgin olive oil
150ml (5fl oz) dry white wine
30g (1oz) butter, melted

Energy 2404kJ/575 Calories, Protein 36.0g,
Total Fat 44.7g, Saturated Fat 12.2g,
Carbohydrate 0.6g, Sugars 0.6g, Dietary
fibre 1.1g, Calcium 46.7mg, Iron 1.5mg.

1. Dry the outside of the chicken with a paper towel or leave uncovered in the fridge for at least an hour.

2. Preheat the oven to 120°C/250°F. Place the chicken in a roasting pan at least 2½cm (1 inch) deep. Using your fingers, gently separate the chicken skin near the breast from the flesh, taking care not to tear the skin.

3. Drizzle the garlic-infused olive oil underneath the skin. Gently push the parsley underneath the skin and season the flesh with a pinch of salt, taking care not to tear the skin.

4. Place the lemon halves, rosemary and thyme in the cavity of the chicken. Tie the legs together with kitchen string.

5. Drizzle the chicken with olive oil, pour the wine around the base and season with salt. Roast the chicken for 1 hour and 30 minutes.

6. Remove the chicken and increase the oven temperature to 220°C/425°F. Brush the melted butter over the chicken and cook for an additional 15–20 minutes or until golden, basting the chicken with the juices from the pan 5–10 minutes before serving.

SERVING SUGGESTION

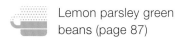 Lemon parsley green beans (page 87)

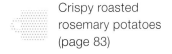 Crispy roasted rosemary potatoes (page 83)

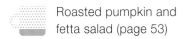 Roasted pumpkin and fetta salad (page 53)

CHICKEN SATAY SKEWERS

SERVES 6

PEANUT SAUCE

3 tbsp crunchy peanut butter

1 tbsp salt reduced soy sauce

1 tbsp lime juice, freshly squeezed

2 tsp brown sugar

1 tsp ginger, finely grated

2–3 tbsp water

SKEWERS

¼ cup coconut milk

2 tbsp salt reduced soy sauce

2½ tsp curry powder

1½ tsp turmeric

1 tbsp brown sugar

1 tbsp grated ginger

1 tbsp fish sauce

600g (1lb 3oz) chicken thigh fillets,
   diced into 3cm (¼ inch) pieces

1 tbsp olive oil

salt and pepper to taste

coriander (cilantro) to serve

spring onions (scallions) (green tops
   only), thinly sliced, to serve

Energy 1530kJ/366 Calories, Protein
19.4g, Total Fat 29.7g, Saturated Fat 9.0g,
Carbohydrate 5.9g, Sugars 4.7g, Dietary
fibre 1.6g, Calcium 31.6mg, Iron 1.9mg.

1. In a small bowl, combine the peanut butter, soy sauce, lime juice, brown sugar and ginger. Add the water and whisk until smooth. Set the peanut sauce aside.

2. In a large bowl, combine the coconut milk, soy sauce, curry powder, turmeric, brown sugar, ginger and fish sauce.

3. Add the diced chicken to the coconut milk mixture, then cover and marinate for 2 hours. Stir occasionally to ensure the chicken is coated in the marinade.

4. Set the grill to medium-high heat. Divide the chicken between skewers, brush with olive oil and season with salt and pepper to taste.

5. Place the skewers onto the hot grill. Grill for approximately 12–25 minutes or until the chicken is cooked, turning the skewers occasionally.

6. Scatter the skewers with coriander and spring onion tops and serve with the peanut sauce.

SERVING SUGGESTION

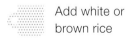 Add white or brown rice

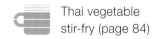 Thai vegetable stir-fry (page 84)

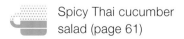 Spicy Thai cucumber salad (page 61)

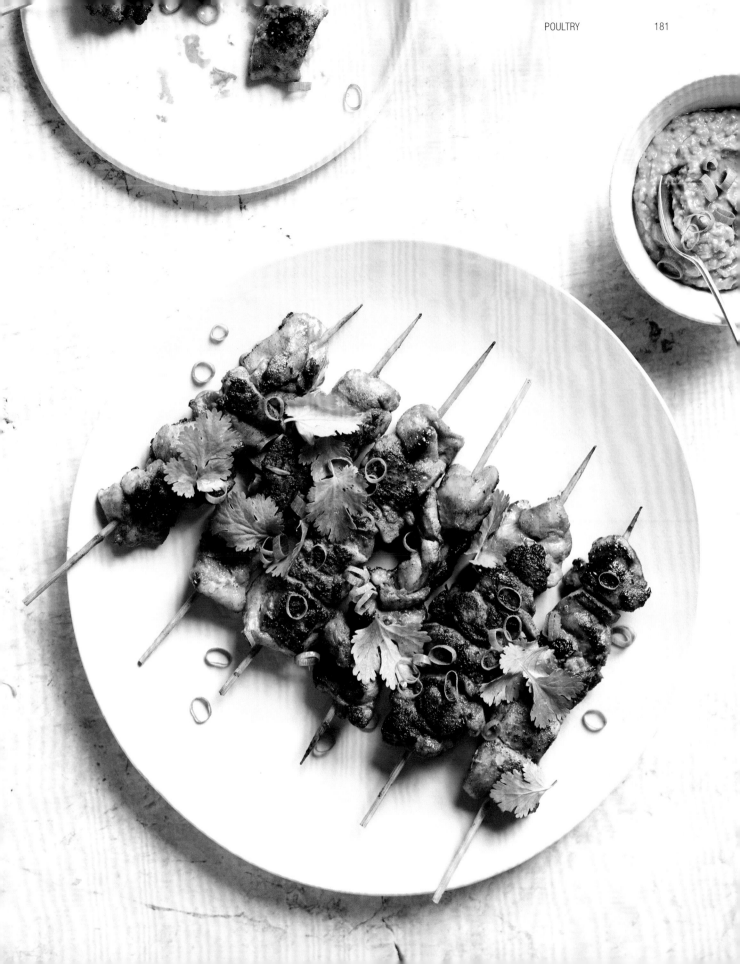

THAI GREEN CHICKEN CURRY

SERVES 4

2 tbsp vegetable oil

2 tbsp low FODMAP green curry paste
(see 'basics', page 234)

400ml (14fl oz) coconut milk

1 tbsp fish sauce

1 tsp brown sugar

5 makrut (kaffir) lime leaves, shredded

700g (1lb 5oz) chicken thigh fillets,
diced into 2.5cm (1 inch) pieces

200g (7oz) eggplant (aubergine), diced
into 1cm (½ inch) pieces

¼ cup Thai basil leaves

Energy 2002kJ/478 Calories, Protein
20.6g, Total Fat 42g, Saturated Fat 17.9g,
Carbohydrate 4.7g, Sugars 4.6g, Dietary
fibre 2.6g, Calcium 44.8mg, Iron 1.8mg.

1. Heat the oil in a large saucepan over medium-high heat.

2. Add the curry paste and stir for 2–3 minutes or until fragrant.

3. Add the coconut milk, fish sauce, brown sugar and lime leaves
and bring to a simmer.

4. Add the chicken pieces, stir, lower the heat to medium and
gently simmer for 6 minutes.

5. Add the diced eggplant (aubergine) and cook for a further 5
minutes or until soft.

6. Stir in half the Thai basil leaves and serve garnished with the
remaining Thai basil.

SERVING SUGGESTION

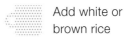 Add white or
brown rice

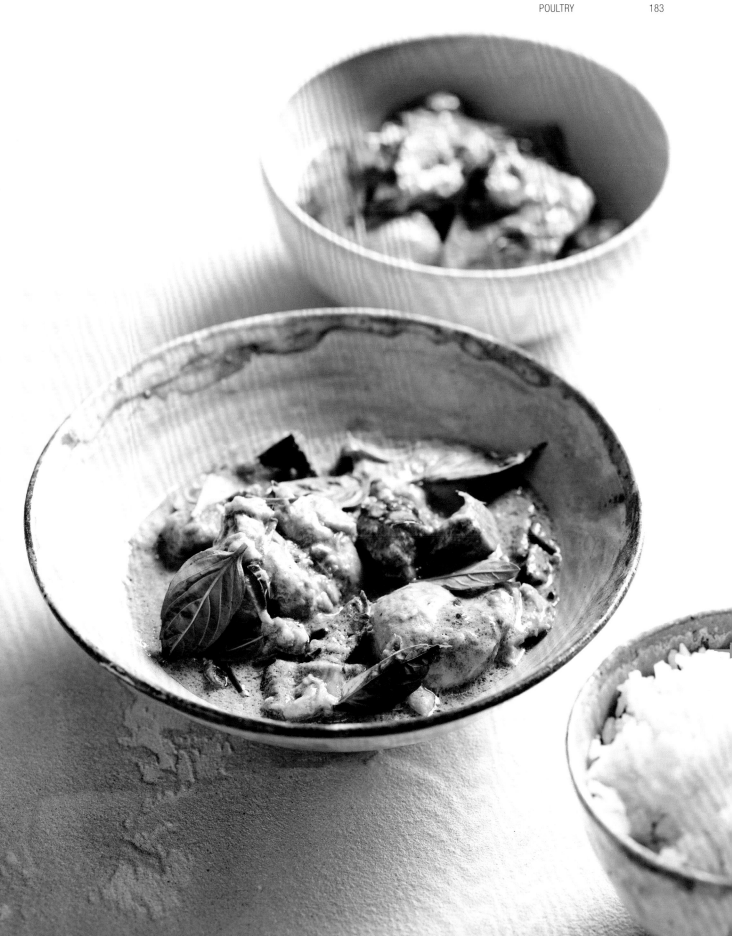

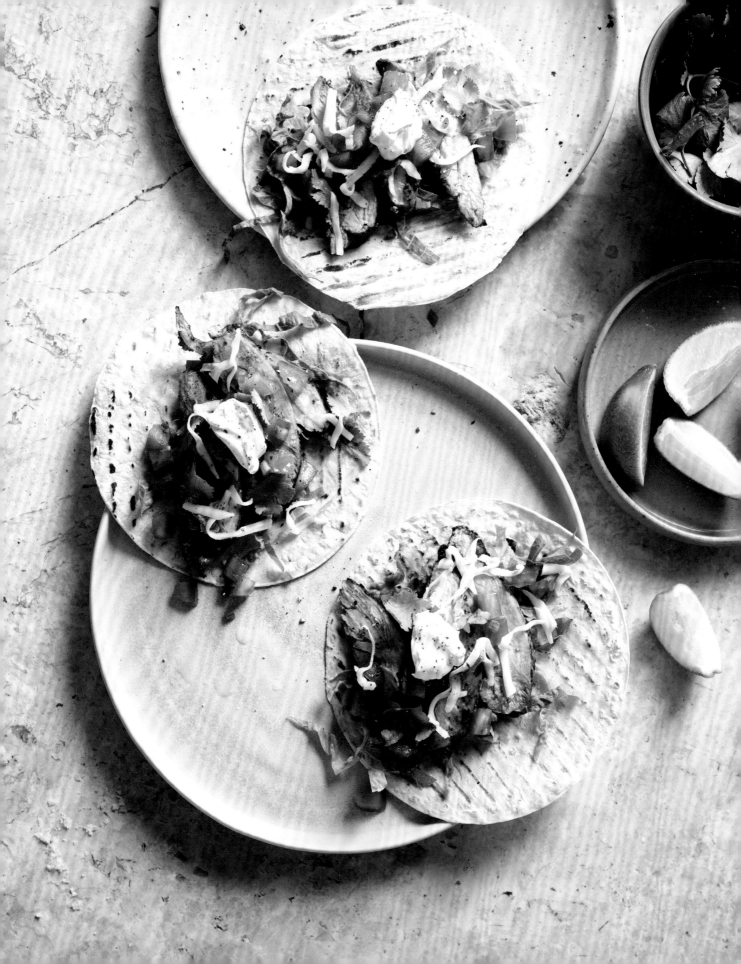

CHICKEN TACOS

SERVES 6

1½ tbsp taco seasoning
 (see 'basics', page 233)

half a lime, juiced

4–5 chicken thigh fillets (about
 1kg/2lb 2oz total)

1 tbsp garlic-infused olive oil

1 cos lettuce, shredded

2 medium-sized tomatoes (common/
 truss), diced

1 jalapeno or to taste, finely chopped

1 cup coriander (cilantro),
 roughly chopped

1 tbsp lime juice

1 cup grated mozzarella

12 corn tortillas

¼ cup sour cream

Energy 2158kJ/516 Calories, Protein
24.1g, Total Fat 23.5g, Saturated Fat 8.0g,
Carbohydrate 49.3g, Sugars 3.9g, Dietary
fibre 4.3g, Calcium 177.7mg, Iron 2.9mg.

1. In a zip lock bag or large bowl, combine the taco seasoning, lime juice and chicken thighs.

2. In a large frypan, heat the garlic-infused olive oil over medium heat. Add the chicken to the pan and cook for 7 minutes on each side or until cooked through.

3. Remove the chicken from the pan, leave it to cool for 5 minutes, then slice thinly and set aside.

4. In a small bowl, combine the diced tomato, jalapeno, coriander (cilantro) and lime juice.

5. Char the tortillas on the stovetop over a gas flame or heat them in a microwave or dry frypan.

6. Divide the chicken among the tortillas and top with lettuce, tomato mixture, cheese and sour cream.

CHICKEN CACCIATORE

SERVES 8

⅓ cup garlic-infused olive oil

1 medium-sized eggplant (aubergine)

2 large carrots

1 cup spring onions (scallions) (green tops only), finely chopped

2 sprigs rosemary

1 tsp dried oregano

1 tsp raw sugar

1 tsp cracked black pepper

1kg (2lb) skinless chicken thighs

250g (9oz) oyster mushrooms, torn into strips

800g (1lb 8oz) tinned whole tomatoes (Roma/plum), diced

1 cup low FODMAP chicken stock

½ cup pitted kalamata olives, halved

1 cup basil or parsley leaves, roughly chopped

Energy 1271kJ/304 Calories, Protein 26.2g, Total Fat 17.3g, Saturated Fat 3.6g, Carbohydrate 8.3g, Sugars 7.8g, Dietary fibre 5.1g, Calcium 86.2mg, Iron 2.8mg.

1. Heat the oil in a large saucepan over high heat. Add the eggplant (aubergine), carrot, spring onion (scallion) tops, rosemary, oregano, sugar and pepper. Cook, stirring occasionally, for approximately 8 minutes or until lightly browned and fragrant.

2. Stir through the chicken pieces, oyster mushrooms, tomato and stock.

3. Cover and cook on medium heat for 20–30 minutes or until the chicken is cooked through and the sauce has thickened slightly. Alternatively, cook in a slow cooker on high heat for 4 hours or on low for 8 hours.

4. Add the halved olives and season with salt.

5. Scatter with basil (or parsley) and serve the cacciatore with mashed potatoes, rice or a low FODMAP pasta.

SERVING SUGGESTION

 Cripsy roasted rosemary potatoes (page 83)

 French green salad (page 51)

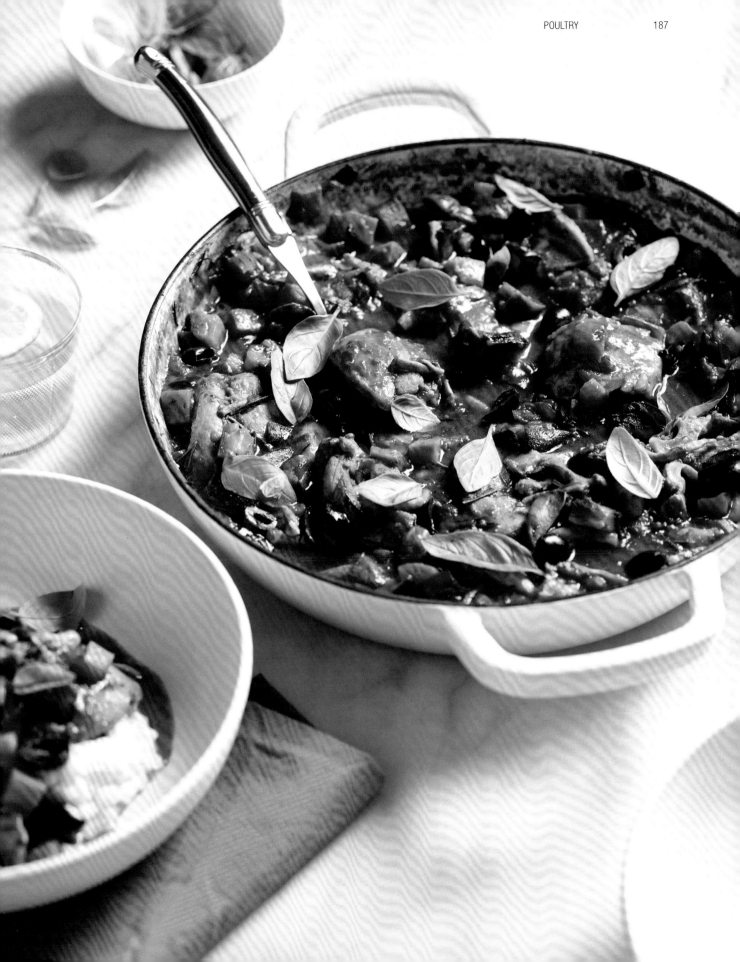

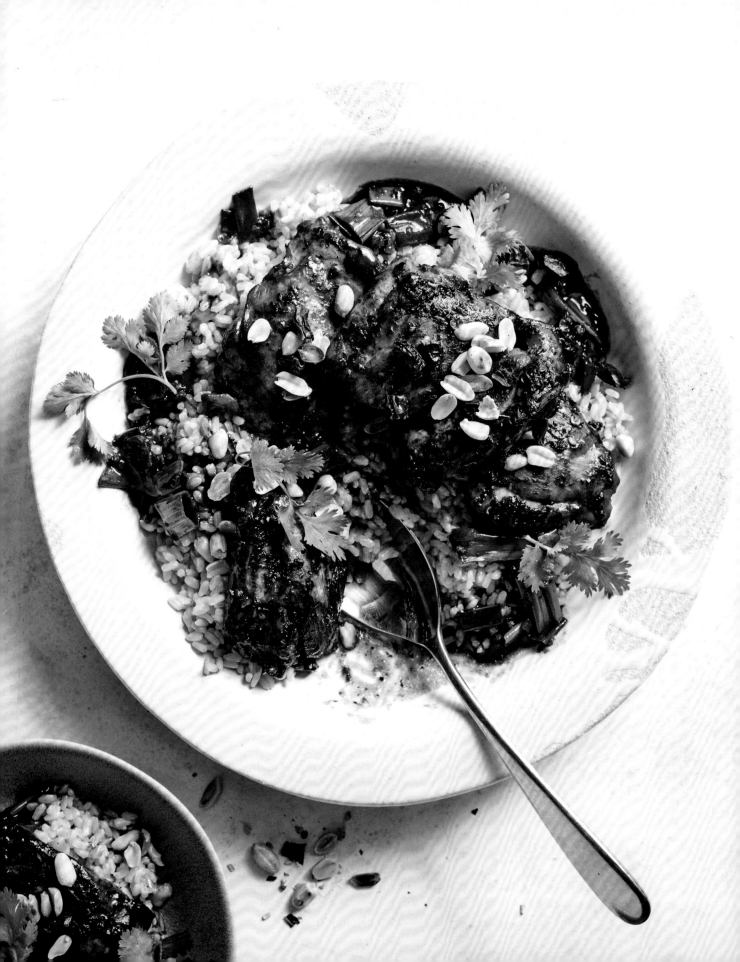

KUNG PAO CHICKEN

SERVES 4

750g (1lb 7oz) chicken thigh fillets

⅓ cup Shaoxing wine

1 tbsp dark soy sauce

4 dried long red chillies,
roughly chopped

1½ tbsp peanut or vegetable oil

3 tsp Sichuan peppercorns,
coarsely crushed

30g (1oz) ginger, skin peeled
and grated

⅓ cup water

¼ cup black Chinese vinegar

2 tbsp light soy sauce

2 tsp cornflour (cornstarch)

1 tsp sesame oil

½ cup spring onions (scallions) (green
tops only), roughly chopped

⅔ cup roasted peanuts

1 cup coriander (cilantro),
roughly chopped

Energy 2124kJ/508 Calories, Protein
40g, Total Fat 35.6g, Saturated Fat 8.2g,
Carbohydrate 4.8g, Sugars 2.1g, Dietary
fibre 3.0g, Calcium 87.4mg, Iron 2.8mg.

1. Place the chicken in a bowl with 2 tbsp Shaoxing wine and the dark soy sauce. Set aside to marinate.

2. Heat a wok over high heat. Add the chillies and stir-fry for approximately 1 minute or until toasted and set aside. Add the oil and Sichuan peppercorns and stir-fry for 1 minute or until fragrant.

3. Add half the ginger and half the marinated chicken and stir-fry for approximately 3-4 minutes or until the chicken is cooked and golden brown. Transfer to a plate and repeat with the remaining ginger and chicken.

4. Prepare the sauce by mixing together the remaining Shaoxing wine, water, vinegar, light soy sauce, cornstarch (cornflour) and sesame oil in a small bowl.

5. Return the chicken to the pan and add the spring onion (scallion) tops and the sauce mixture. Bring to the boil over high heat.

6. Add the peanuts and toasted chillies and toss to combine. Scatter the chicken with spring onion tops and coriander (cilantro) and serve with rice.

SERVING SUGGESTION

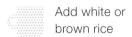 Add white or
brown rice

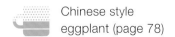 Chinese style
eggplant (page 78)

SUMAC ROASTED CHICKEN WITH POLENTA

SERVES 4

1 small chicken, skin on, cut into 4–6
  pieces (1–1.2kg/2lb–2lb 6oz)
¼ cup lemon juice
¼ cup garlic-infused olive oil
¼ cup sumac
½ tsp ground cumin
½ tsp cinnamon
salt and pepper to taste
1 tbsp extra virgin olive oil
1 cup polenta
4 cup low FODMAP chicken stock or
  water
3 tsp butter
¼ cup pine nuts
¼ cup parsley, roughly chopped
¼ cup spring onions (scallions) (green
  tops only), roughly chopped
coriander (cilantro) to serve

Energy 3068kJ/733 Calories, Protein
57.9g, Total Fat 39.4g, Saturated Fat 7.3g,
Carbohydrate 35.7g, Sugars 1.3g, Dietary
fibre 3.5g, Calcium 57.7mg, Iron 3.9mg.

1. Slash the flesh of each piece of chicken, making diagonal cuts approximately 2cm (¾ inch) apart. Place the meat in a large bowl.

2. Combine the lemon juice, garlic-infused olive oil, sumac, cumin, cinnamon, and salt and pepper to taste. Rub the mixture into the meat. Cover and transfer to the refrigerator to marinate for 1–6 hours.

3. Preheat the oven to 220°C/425°F.

4. Heat the olive oil in a large ovenproof frypan over high heat. Remove the chicken from the marinade, add it to the pan and cook, turning frequently, until brown all over.

5. Pour the marinade over the chicken, then transfer the pan to the oven and cook for 30 minutes, turning the chicken after 15 minutes.

6. Meanwhile, prepare the polenta. Place the chicken stock or water in a small saucepan and bring to a simmer over medium heat. Add the polenta and whisk continuously, until the mixture returns to a simmer. Reduce the heat to low and cook, stirring often, for 10–15 minutes or until the polenta is cooked through. Stir in the butter and set the polenta aside.

7. Toast the pine nuts by placing them in a small pan over medium-low heat. Stir for 2-3 minutes or until browned.

8. Pour the polenta onto a serving dish and arrange the chicken on top. Garnish with spring onion (scallions) tops, parsley and pine nuts.

SERVING SUGGESTION

 Tabouli (page 64)

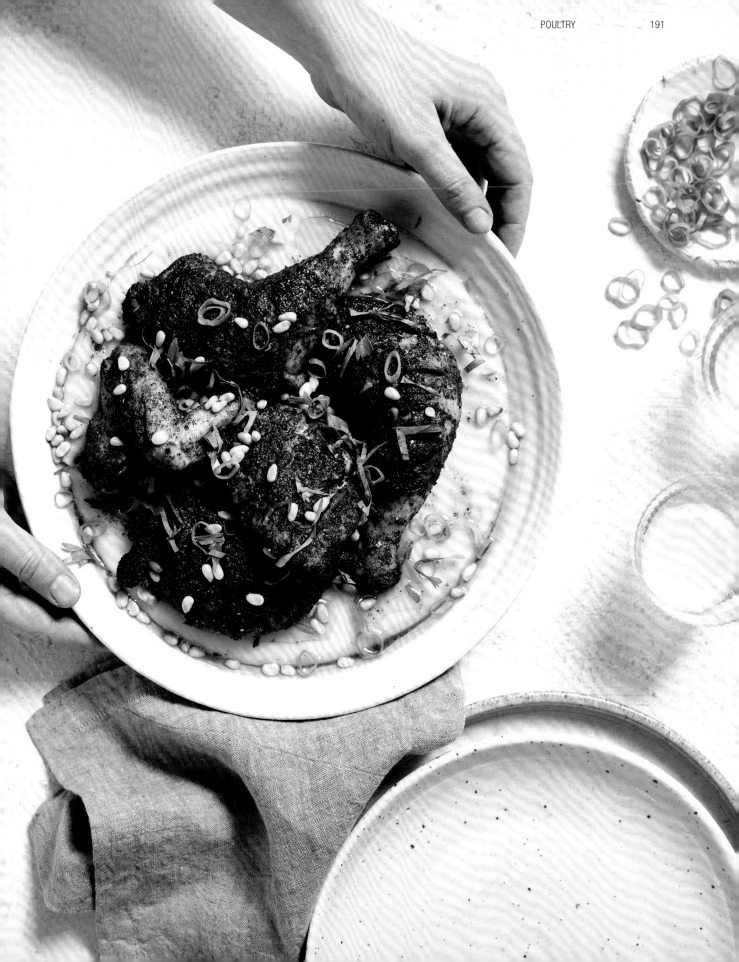

INDIAN CHICKEN CURRY WITH COCONUT MILK

SERVES 6

1½ kg (3lb) chicken, cut into pieces
2 tbsp olive oil (garlic-infused or plain)
¼ tsp fenugreek seeds
10 fresh curry leaves
1 cup spring onions (scallions) (green
   top only), finely chopped
2 tsp finely grated ginger
½ tsp chilli flakes
1 tsp ground turmeric
1 tbsp ground coriander
1 tsp ground cumin
½ tsp fennel seeds
2 tsp paprika
½ tsp salt or to taste
2 tbsp white wine vinegar
2 medium-sized tomatoes (common/
   truss), finely chopped
4 cardamon pods, bruised
2 strips lemon rind (without white pith)
200ml (7fl oz) coconut milk (fat
   reduced or full fat)
1 tbsp lemon juice
½ cup basil or coriander
   (cilantro) leaves

1. Chop the chicken into eight pieces, or ask a butcher to do it for you.

2. Heat the oil in a heavy-based pot or casserole over low heat.

3. Add the curry leaves and fenugreek seeds and fry until they begin to brown. Take care not to burn them.

4. Add the spring onion (scallion) tops and ginger and stir for 1–2 minutes or until wilted.

5. Add the chilli, turmeric, coriander, cumin, fennel seeds, paprika, salt and vinegar. Stir well.

6. Increase the heat to medium and add the chicken pieces, turning them to coat them well with the spices. Add the chopped tomatoes, cardamom pods and lemon rind.

7. Cover the pot with a lid and simmer over low heat for 40–50 minutes, stirring occasionally, until the chicken is tender.

8. Remove the pan from the heat and stir in the coconut milk and lemon juice.

9. Serve sprinkled with basil or coriander leaves.

Energy 1854kJ/443 Calories, Protein
51g, Total Fat 24.6g, Saturated Fat 7.5g,
Carbohydrate 3.3g, Sugars 2.2g, Dietary
fibre 1.7g, Calcium 51.1mg, Iron 2.7mg.

SERVING SUGGESTION

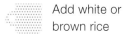 Add white or
brown rice

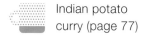 Indian potato
curry (page 77)

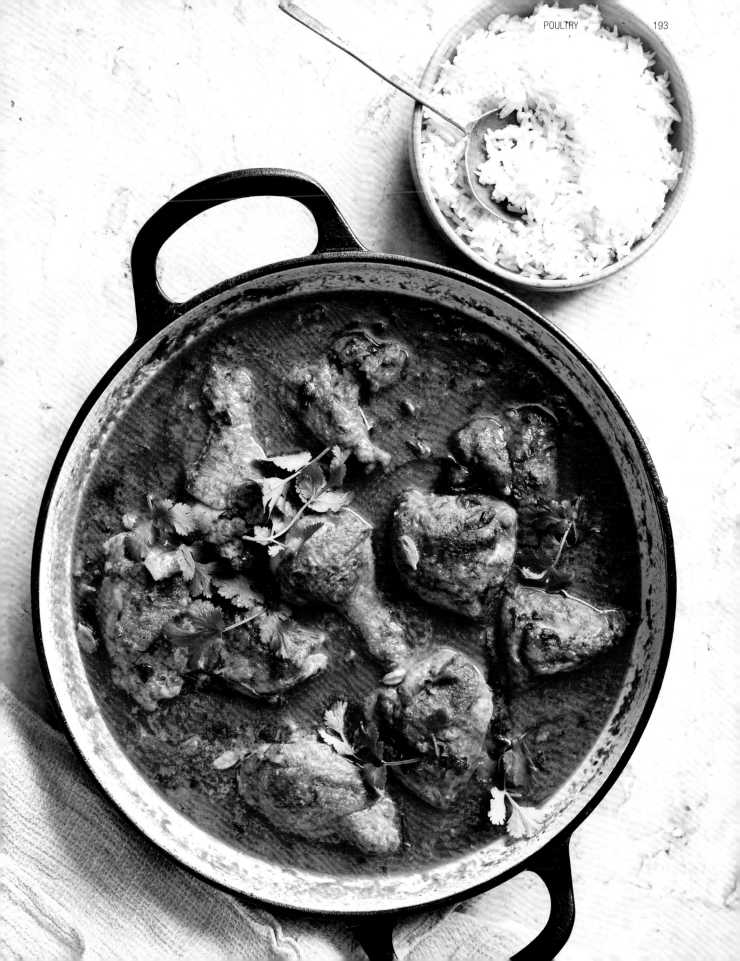

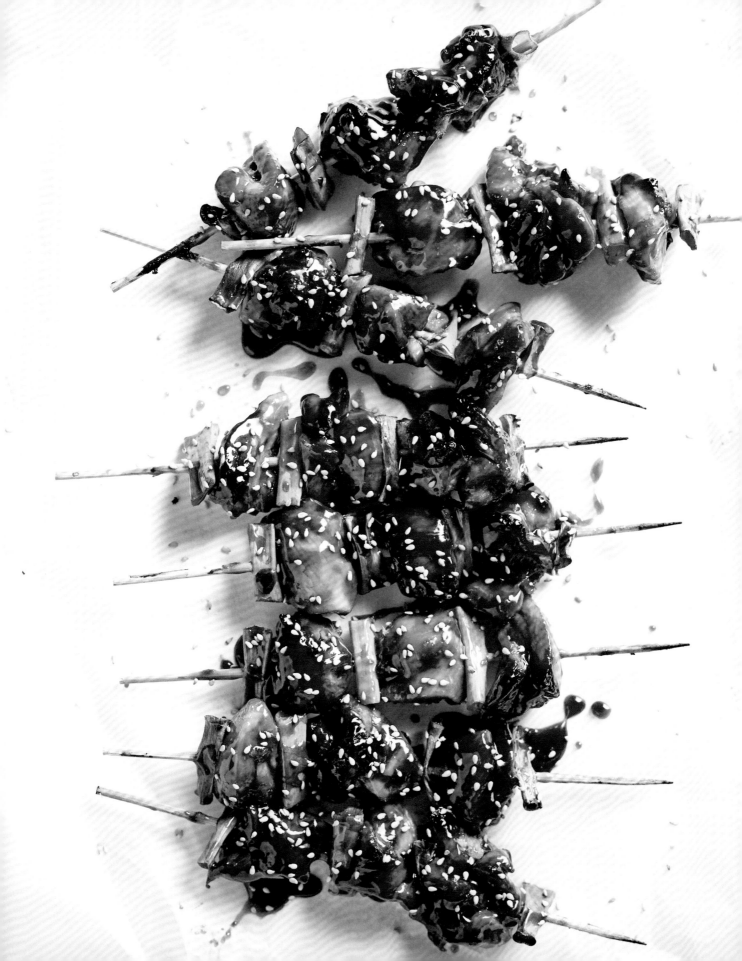

CHICKEN YAKITORI

SERVES 4

12 bamboo skewers

650g (1lb 4oz) chicken thigh fillets

½ cup spring onions (scallions) (green tops only)

1 tbsp sesame seeds

SAUCE

1½ tsp cornflour (cornstarch)

½ tbsp cold water

½ cup soy sauce

½ cup mirin

¼ cup Chinese rice wine

¼ cup water

1 tbsp brown sugar

1 thumb-sized piece of ginger

Energy 1528kJ/365 Calories, Protein 31.2g, Total Fat 15.2g, Saturated Fat 4.3g, Carbohydrate 19.4g, Sugars 16.4g, Dietary fibre 0.9g, Calcium 34.9mg, Iron 2.0mg.

1. Soak the bamboo skewers in water for approximately 20 minutes.

2. To make the yakitori sauce, combine the cornflour (cornstarch) and water in a small bowl and set aside. Combine all the other sauce ingredients in a small saucepan and bring to a boil over medium heat. Reduce the heat to low and simmer uncovered until the sauce reduces by a quarter.

3. Remove the ginger from the saucepan (discard) and mix in the cornflour mixture. Bring back to the boil and cook for 1–2 minutes or until the sauce thickens.

4. Cut the chicken thighs into 3cm (1¼ inch) pieces.

5. Slice the spring onion (scallion) tops into 3cm (1¼ inch) lengths and thread the chicken and spring onions onto the skewers.

6. Turn the oven grill to high heat and place the skewers onto a baking tray. Using a pastry brush, lightly coat the skewers with the sauce. Place them under the grill.

7. Cook the skewers for 15 minutes or until they are cooked through and caramelised, turning them and brushing them with more sauce every few minutes.

8. Remove the skewers from the grill and brush them once more with sauce. Sprinkle with sesame seeds to serve.

SERVING SUGGESTION

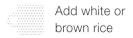 Add white or brown rice

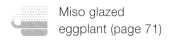 Miso glazed eggplant (page 71)

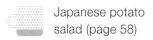 Japanese potato salad (page 58)

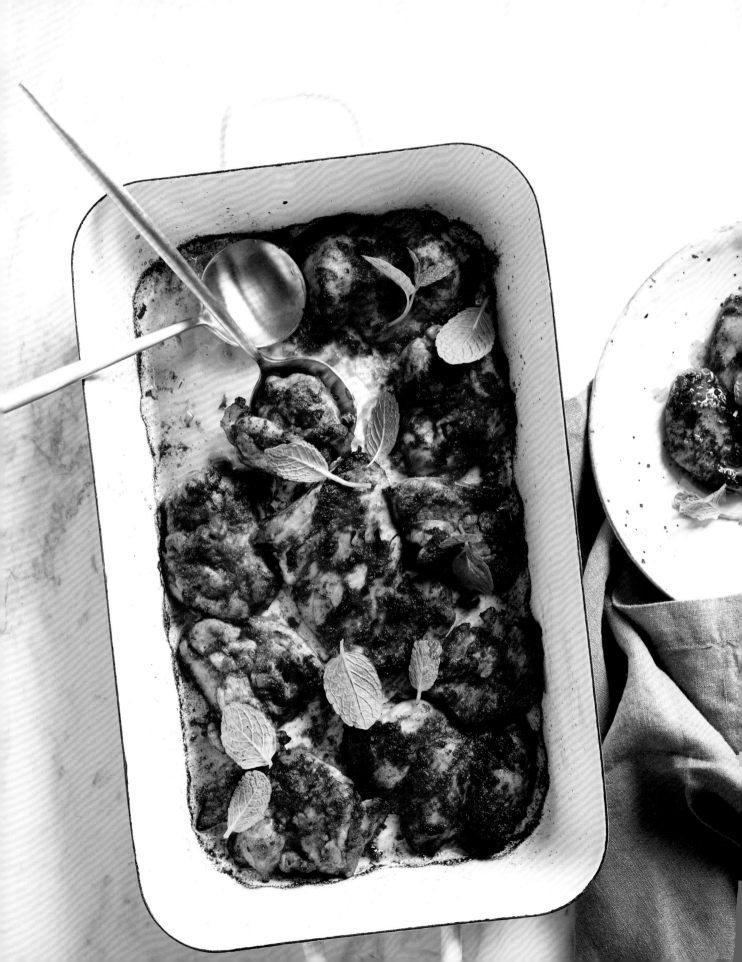

TANDOORI CHICKEN

SERVES 5

5 skinless chicken thigh fillets
(750g/1lb 7oz), cut into 2 pieces
½ tsp saffron strands
1 tbsp boiling water
1 tbsp grated ginger
1 tbsp lemon juice
½ tsp dried crushed red chilli, or
to taste
1 tsp paprika
salt to taste
2 tbsp oil (garlic-infused or plain)
2 tbsp mint leaves

Energy 894kJ/214 Calories, Protein 26.7g,
Total Fat 11.6g, Saturated Fat 2.4g,
Carbohydrate 0.3g, Sugars 0.2g, Dietary
fibre 0.5g, Calcium 17.8mg, Iron 0.9 mg.

1. Dry the chicken with a paper towel and make slits in the flesh. Set aside.

2. Soak the saffron in the boiling water for 10–15 minutes.

3. To make the spice mixture, place the soaked saffron and water in a spice blender and add the grated ginger, lemon juice, dried crushed chillies, paprika and salt. Blend well.

4. Rub the spice mixture into the chicken pieces. Cover, refrigerate and leave to marinate for at least 2 hours and preferably overnight. Allowing the chicken to marinate overnight will produce a stronger flavour.

5. Preheat the oven to 180°C/350°F. Line a large tray with foil and place the marinated chicken pieces on a rack in the tray (reserve the marinade). Brush the chicken pieces with the remaining garlic-infused oil. Bake the chicken for 20 minutes. Turn the chicken over and brush with marinade and oil. Bake for a further 20 minutes or until well cooked.

6. Scatter with mint leaves and serve.

SERVING SUGGESTION

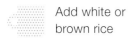 Add white or brown rice

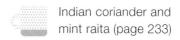 Indian coriander and mint raita (page 233)

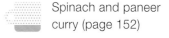 Spinach and paneer curry (page 152)

CHICKEN PROVENÇALE

SERVES 6

1 whole chicken, cut into 8 pieces
  (1.8 kg/4lb)
160g (5½oz) red capsicum (bell
  pepper), chargrilled
160g (5½oz) green capsicum (bell
  pepper), chargrilled
400g (14oz) canned tomatoes
2 small zucchinis (courgettes)
2 anchovies, finely chopped
½ cup black kalamata olives, pitted
2 tbsp parsley, chopped
2 tbsp garlic-infused olive oil
1 cup finely chopped spring onions
  (scallions), green tops only
½ cup dry white wine
½ cup low FODMAP chicken stock
1 thyme sprig
1 bay leaf
¼ tsp black pepper, ground
salt to taste

Energy 1703kJ/407 Calories, Protein
29.4g, Total Fat 27.6g, Saturated Fat 7.1g,
Carbohydrate 5.6g, Sugars 5.4g, Dietary
fibre 2.6g, Calcium 54.6mg, Iron 2.1mg.

1. Preheat the oven to 180°C/350°F. Dry the chicken pieces with absorbent paper.

2. Chop the chargrilled capsicums (bell peppers) and zucchinis into large pieces. Finely chop the canned tomatoes and set aside.

3. Place the anchovies in a small bowl over a saucepan of simmering water and stir occasionally until the anchovies dissolve. Remove the bowl from the heat and add the olives and chopped parsley. Stir well and set aside.

4. Preheat a large heavy-based casserole dish with a well-fitting lid over medium-high heat. Add the oil and brown the chicken pieces in batches. Transfer the cooked chicken pieces to a dish and set aside.

5. Reduce the heat and add the finely chopped spring onion (scallion) tops and cook for 2–3 minutes or until wilted. Arrange the cooked chicken pieces (including meat juices) in the casserole dish, add the wine and chicken stock and simmer for 2–3 minutes. Stir in the chopped tomatoes, thyme sprig and bay leaf. Cover with a lid, transfer carefully to the oven and cook for 45 minutes.

6. Remove the casserole from the oven and carefully stir in the capsicum and zucchini. Add the black pepper and salt to taste. Return to the oven for an additional 20 minutes.

7. Scatter with the anchovy, olive and parsley mixture and serve.

SERVING SUGGESTION

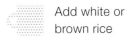 Add white or brown rice

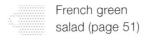 French green salad (page 51)

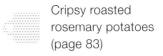 Cripsy roasted rosemary potatoes (page 83)

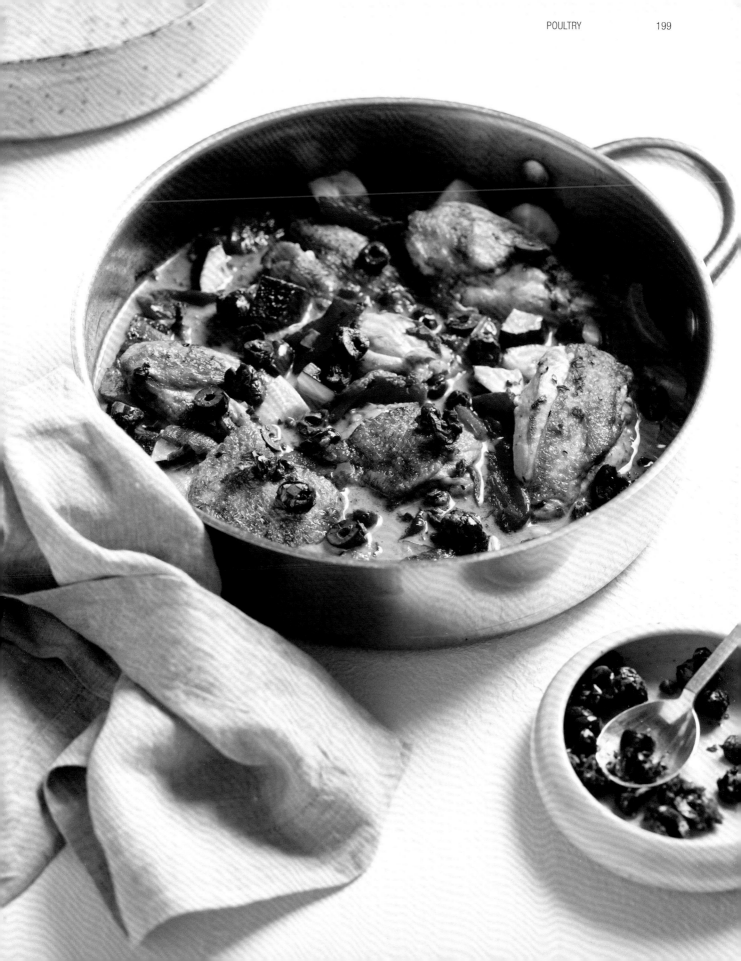

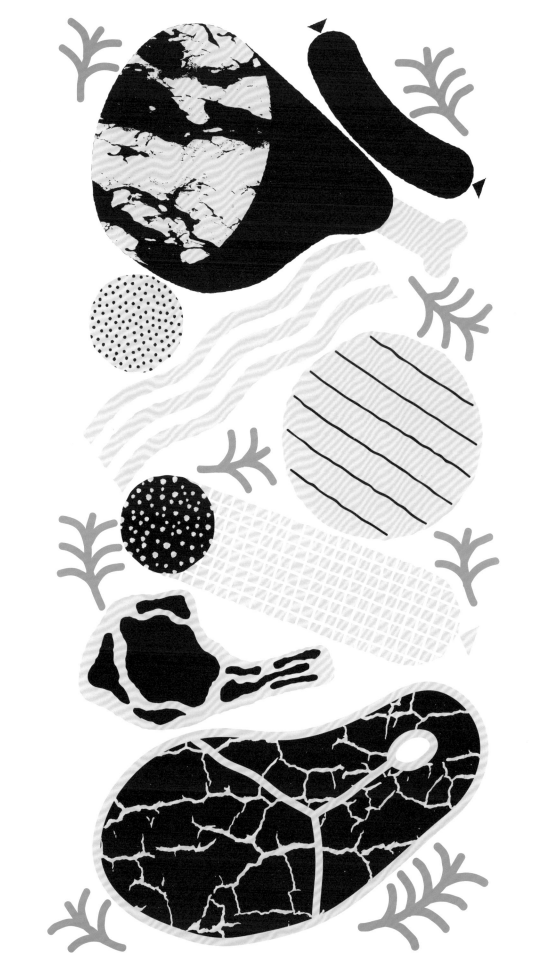

RED MEAT

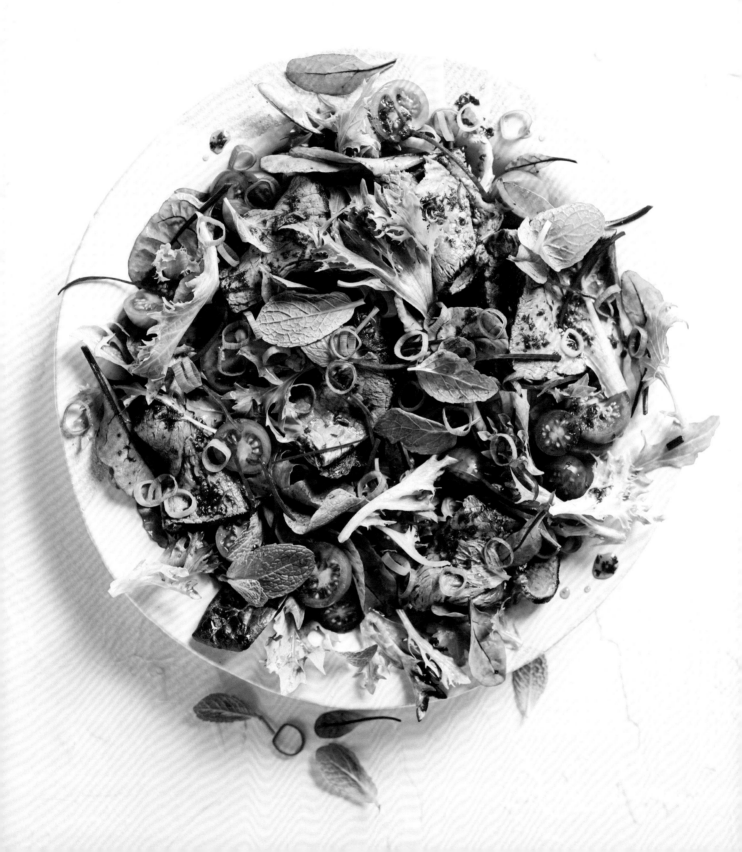

THAI BEEF SALAD

SERVES 5

750g (1lb 6oz) lean beef steak
   (sirloin, rump or fillet)
1 tbsp garlic-infused oil (or plain)
½ cup coriander (cilantro)
   leaves, chopped
2 tbsp soy sauce
2 tbsp fresh lime juice or lemon juice
1 tbsp fish sauce
1½ tbsp palm sugar
1 cos (romaine) lettuce, leaves
   separated, or 200g (7oz) mixed
   salad leaves
½ cup spring onions (scallions) (green
   tops only), finely chopped
1–2 fresh red chillies, cut into strips
250g (9oz) cherry tomatoes, halved
¼ cup mint leaves

Energy 1195kJ/286 Calories, Protein
36.6g, Total Fat 12.1g, Saturated Fat 3.9g,
Carbohydrate 5.9g, Sugars 5.5g, Dietary
fibre 2.8g, Calcium 40.5mg, Iron 4.4mg.

1. Cook the beef to your liking (medium-rare, medium or well-done) in a hot pan with the garlic-infused oil.

2. Remove the beef from the pan and set aside to cool.

3. To prepare the dressing, combine the chopped coriander (cilantro) leaves, soy sauce, lime juice, fish sauce and sugar in a spice blender. Blitz until the sugar has dissolved and the mixture is well combined.

4. Slice the beef thinly and place in a bowl.

5. Pour the dressing over the beef and toss gently to coat the beef.

6. Arrange the lettuce leaves on a serving platter.

7. Layer the sliced beef over the lettuce. Sprinkle over the spring onion (scallion) tops, chilli, cherry tomatoes and fresh mint leaves and serve.

SERVING SUGGESTION

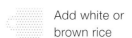

Add white or
brown rice

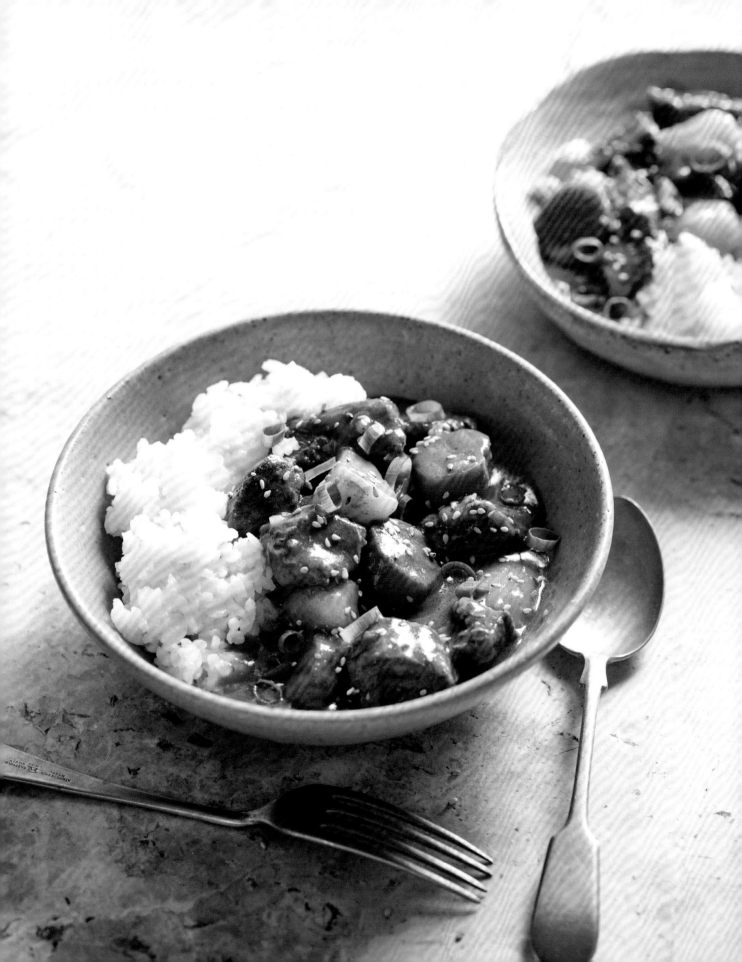

JAPANESE BEEF CURRY

SERVES 6

2 tsp olive oil

1 tbsp butter

1kg (2lb) chuck steak, cut into cubes

1 tbsp grated ginger

2 tbsp garlic-infused olive oil

2 tbsp curry powder

2 tsp garam masala

¼ cup gluten-free flour

3 cups low FODMAP beef stock

2 potatoes, peeled and cut into cubes

2 tsp apple cider vinegar

1 large carrot, peeled and chopped

1 tbsp tomato sauce (low
    FODMAP ketchup)

1 tbsp Worcestershire sauce

1 tbsp soy sauce

white rice to serve

1 tbsp toasted sesame seeds to serve

¼ cup spring onions (scallions) (green
    tops only) to serve, thinly sliced

Energy 1902kJ/455 Calories, Protein
40.2g, Total Fat 24.6g, Saturated Fat 7.3g,
Carbohydrate 16.8g, Sugars 3.7g, Dietary
fibre 3.4g, Calcium 46.6mg, Iron 4.4mg.

1. In a large heavy-based pot, heat the oil and butter over high heat. Season the meat and cook in batches for approximately 5 minutes or until brown. Place the beef on a plate and set aside.

2. Turn the heat to low. Add the ginger and garlic-infused olive oil to the pot and cook for 1 minute. Stir in the curry powder and garam masala.

3. Return the meat to the pot and increase the heat to high. Add the flour and stir until the beef is coated. Add the low FODMAP beef stock and mix until the curry is smooth.

4. Add the potato, carrot, and apple cider vinegar to the pot and bring to a boil. Set the heat to low.

5. Cover the pot with a lid and simmer for 2 hours or until the meat is tender.

6. Remove from the heat and add the tomato sauce (low FODMAP ketchup), Worcestershire sauce, and soy sauce to the pot. Allow to rest for 10 minutes.

7. Serve over steamed rice. Sprinkle over sesame seeds and green spring onion (scallion) tops.

SERVING SUGGESTION

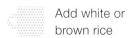 Add white or brown rice

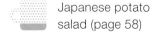 Japanese potato salad (page 58)

SPAGHETTI BOLOGNESE

SERVES 6

1 tbsp garlic-infused olive oil

1 cup spring onions (scallions) (green tops only), chopped

2 thin slices of pancetta, chopped

2 fresh sprigs of rosemary

3 medium-sized carrots, peeled and finely chopped

500g (1lb) lean beef mince

1 tbsp tomato paste

400g (14oz) tinned whole tomatoes (Roma/plum), chopped

1 tsp balsamic vinegar

1 low FODMAP beef stock cube, crumbled

400ml (14fl oz) boiling water

2 dried bay leaves

cracked black pepper to taste

500g (1lb) gluten-free spaghetti

⅓ cup grated parmesan

Energy 2349kJ/561 Calories, Protein 31.0g, Total Fat 16.2g, Saturated Fat 6.9g, Carbohydrate 71.3g, Sugars 9.0g, Dietary fibre 5.9g, Calcium 133.5mg, Iron 3.8mg.

1. Heat the garlic-infused olive oil in a large, non-stick pan on medium-high heat.

2. Add the spring onion (scallion) tops and cook for 5 minutes or until soft and slightly browned.

3. Add the pancetta and rosemary and cook for a further 5-10 minutes or until the pancetta starts to brown.

4. Add the carrot, then cook with the lid on for 10-15 minutes, stirring occasionally, until the vegetables are soft and slightly brown.

5. Increase the heat to high and add the beef mince. Cook for 10 minutes, stirring often to break up any lumps.

6. Add the tomato paste, tinned tomatoes, balsamic vinegar and bay leaves.

7. Add the stock cube and water, stirring well until combined.

8. Cover, bring to the boil, then reduce heat to a simmer and cook for 1 hour, stirring occasionally.

9. Remove lid and continue to cook for 15 minutes to reduce sauce slightly.

10. Boil water for the pasta and cook according to packet directions.

11. Remove bay leaves from sauce, then serve sauce with cooked spaghetti and a sprinkle of parmesan cheese.

SERVING SUGGESTION

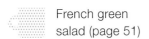
French green salad (page 51)

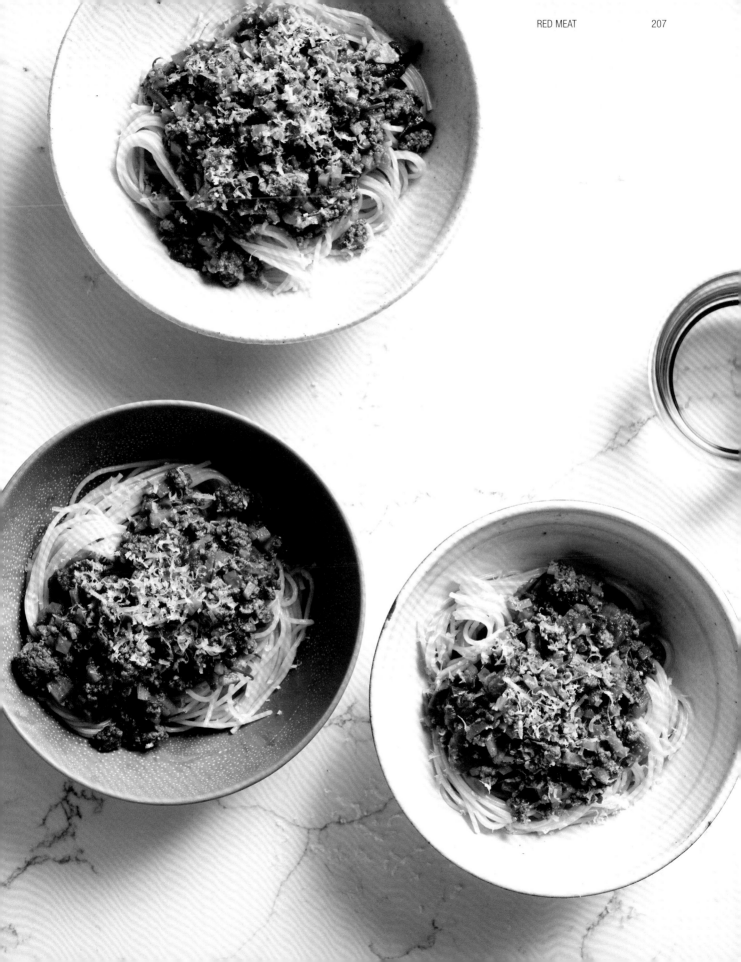

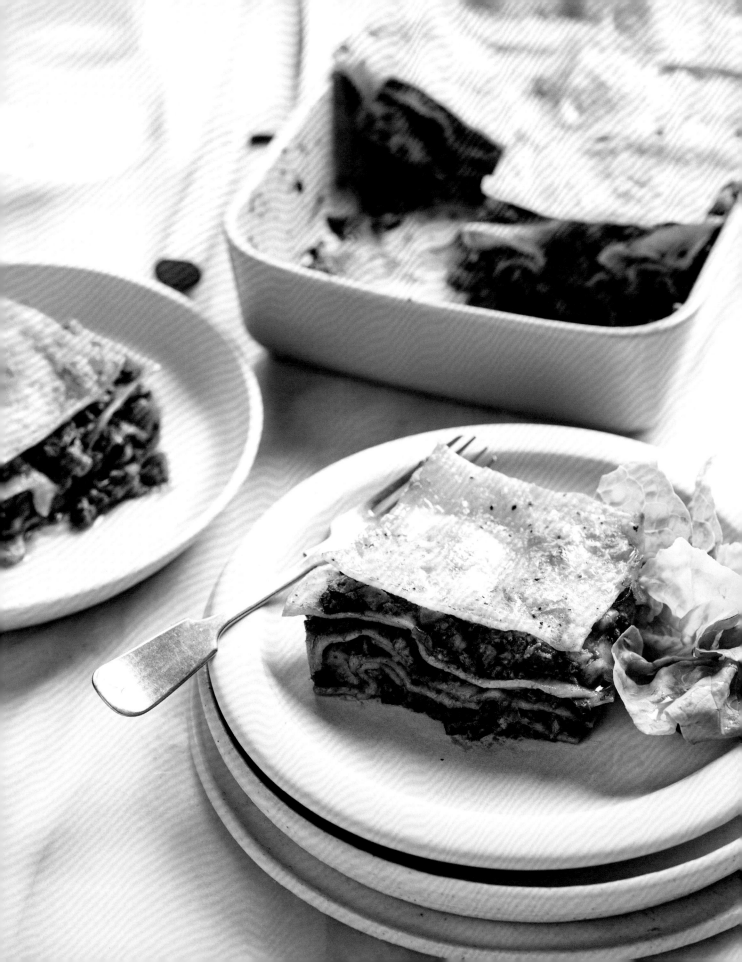

LASAGNE

SERVES 8

1 quantity bolognese sauce (see
   page 206)
450ml (15fl oz) light cooking cream
   (lactose free if required)
250g (9oz) parmesan, shaved
350g (12oz) gluten-free
   lasagne sheets

Energy 2302kJ/550 Calories, Protein 29.2g,
Total Fat 29.6g, Saturated Fat 17.1g,
Carbohydrate 40.0g, Sugars 6.4g, Dietary
fibre 3.0g, Calcium 404.7mg, Iron 2.1mg.

1. Preheat the oven to 180°C/350°F.

2. Divide the bolognese sauce into portions: for this recipe you
   will need only two-thirds of the sauce. Freeze the remaining
   one-third for an easy midweek meal.

3. Spread a quarter of the sauce you are using into the base of a
   deep oven-safe dish, approximately 25cm x 30cm (10 inches
   x 12 inches). Top with a single layer of lasagne sheets.

4. Pour a quarter of the cream over the lasagne sheets and
   spread evenly. Sprinkle with a quarter of the parmesan cheese.
   Repeat these layers three more times, each time layering the
   bolognese sauce, lasagne sheets, cream and parmesan.

5. Bake the lasagne for 45 minutes, or until the lasagne sheets are
   soft when you test the middle of the dish with a knife.

6. Serve with a green salad (see page 51).

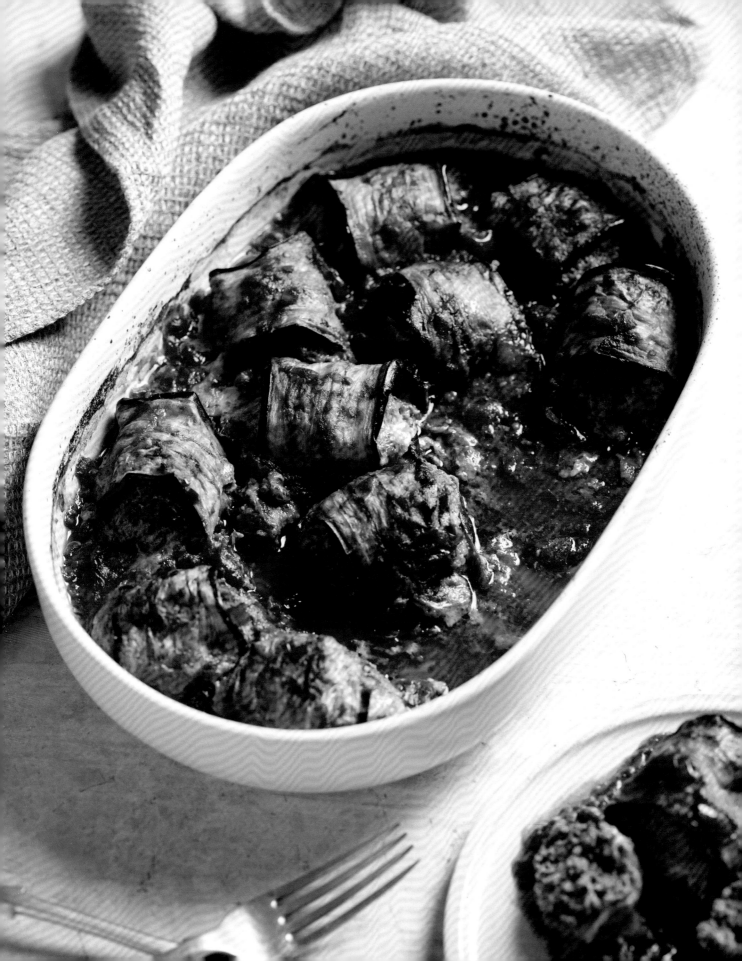

MIDDLE EASTERN BAKED KOFTAS

SERVES 4

2 medium-sized eggplants
   (aubergines)
2 tbsp garlic-infused oil
700g (1lb 5oz) minced beef
   (ground beef)
1 cup finely chopped parsley
1½ tsp cinnamon
1 tsp allspice
1 tsp chilli powder
1 egg, whisked
salt and pepper to taste

TOMATO SAUCE

1 tbsp extra virgin olive oil
2 tbsp garlic-infused olive oil
400g (14oz) tinned whole tomatoes
   (Roma/plum), chopped
¼ cup water
½ tsp chilli flakes

Energy 2688kJ/642 Calories, Protein 43.7g,
Total Fat 47.6g, Saturated Fat 13.1g,
Carbohydrate 9.0g, Sugars 7.2g, Dietary
fibre 5.3g, Calcium 89mg, Iron 4.2mg.

1. Preheat the oven to 220°C/425°F.

2. Cut the eggplant (aubergine) lengthways into long, wide slices about ½cm (¼ inch) thick. Brush each side with garlic-infused olive oil and bake for 15 minutes or until slightly golden.

3. Mix the minced beef (ground beef) with the allspice, chilli powder, parsley, egg, cinnamon, salt and pepper using either your hands or a food processor until well combined.

4. Divide the mixture into 12 equal portions and mould into oval shapes. Set aside in the refrigerator.

5. To make the tomato sauce, add the oils to a medium-sized saucepan or frypan and place on a medium-high heat. Add the tomatoes, water and chilli. Bring to a boil and then reduce the heat to medium-low. Cook the sauce for 10 minutes or until thick.

6. Roll each kofta up in a slice of eggplant and place into a large baking dish, seam side down. Pour the tomato sauce over the top of the koftas, cover the dish tightly with foil and bake for 20 minutes. Remove from the foil and cook for another 15 minutes, then serve.

SERVING SUGGESTION

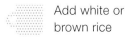
Add white or
brown rice

LAMB ROGAN JOSH

SERVES 6

750g (1lb 6oz) lean lamb

1 tsp crushed red chillies

2 tbsp desiccated coconut

1 tbsp ground coriander

1 tsp ground cumin

1 tsp poppy seeds

½ tsp fennel seeds

2 tbsp water

¼ cup garlic-infused or plain olive oil

1 cup spring onions (scallions) (green tops only), finely chopped

1 tbsp finely grated ginger

½ cup coriander (cilantro) leaves, chopped

½ tsp turmeric

4 cardamom pods, bruised

½ cup plain lactose-free yoghurt

2 medium-sized tomatoes (common/truss), finely chopped

½ tsp salt, or to taste

¼ tsp black pepper, or to taste

1 tsp garam masala

¼ cup coriander (cilantro) leaves, extra, for serving

Energy 1258kJ/300 Calories, Protein 29.4g, Total Fat 17.2g, Saturated Fat 5.0g, Carbohydrate 6.0g, Sugars 4.3g, Dietary fibre 3.0g, Calcium 83mg, Iron 4.5mg.

1. Cut the lamb into cubes.

2. Heat a dry frypan over a medium heat, add crushed red chillies, desiccated coconut, gound coriander, cumin, poppy seeds and fennel seeds. Shake the pan until the coconut has roasted. Remove from heat and add to a small spice blender.

3. Add the water to the spice blender and blend for a few seconds or until smooth.

4. Heat the oil in a heavy-based pot or casserole over low heat and fry the chopped spring onion (scallion) tops, grated ginger and coriander leaves for a few minutes while stirring. Add the turmeric, bruised cardamom pods and spice mixture and stir. Add the yoghurt, chopped tomatoes and salt and pepper, and stir for a further 5 minutes.

5. Increase the heat to medium, add the lamb and stir to coat it with the spices. Reduce the heat to low, cover the pot with a lid and cook for 55 minutes or until the lamb is tender, stirring occasionally.

6. Stir in the garam masala and cook for a further 5 minutes. Serve scattered with coriander leaves.

SERVING SUGGESTION

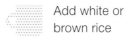 Add white or brown rice

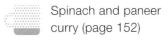 Spinach and paneer curry (page 152)

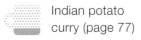 Indian potato curry (page 77)

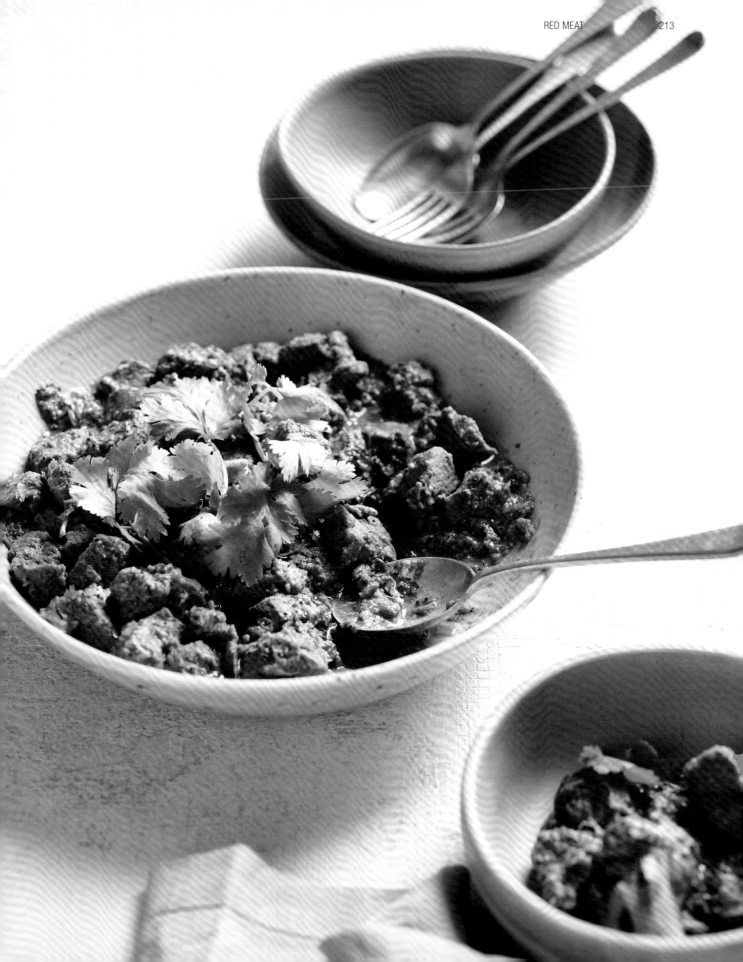

FRENCH LAMB SHANKS

SERVES 6

6 lamb shanks

2 tbsp garlic-infused

1 cup spring onions (scallions) (green tops only), finely chopped

½ cup tomato paste

1 cup low FODMAP beef stock

½ cup red wine

salt and pepper to taste

½ cup parsley, chopped

Energy 2545kJ/608 Calories, Protein 47.7g, Total Fat 43.9g, Saturated Fat 16.0g, Carbohydrate 2.2g, Sugars 2.0g, Dietary fibre 0.8g, Calcium 35.1mg, Iron 3.9mg.

1. Dry the lamb shanks with paper towel. Preheat the oven to 160°C/320°F.

2. Heat the oil in a heavy-based casserole dish with a well-fitted lid and cook the lamb shanks in batches over medium heat until all shanks are lightly browned. Turn frequently. Remove from the casserole dish and set aside.

3. Reduce the heat to low and add the chopped spring onion (scallion) tops. Cook for 3-5 minutes or until wilted.

4. Return the browned lamb shanks to the casserole dish, and add the tomato paste, beef stock and red wine. Stir well to combine the ingredients and coat the lamb shanks with sauce.

5. Transfer the dish to the oven and cook, turning the shanks occasionally, for 2 hours or until the meat is very tender and falling from the bone.

6. Sprinkle with chopped parsley to serve.

SERVING SUGGESTION

 Cripsy roasted rosemary potatoes (page 83)

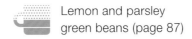 Lemon and parsley green beans (page 87)

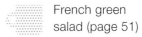 French green salad (page 51)

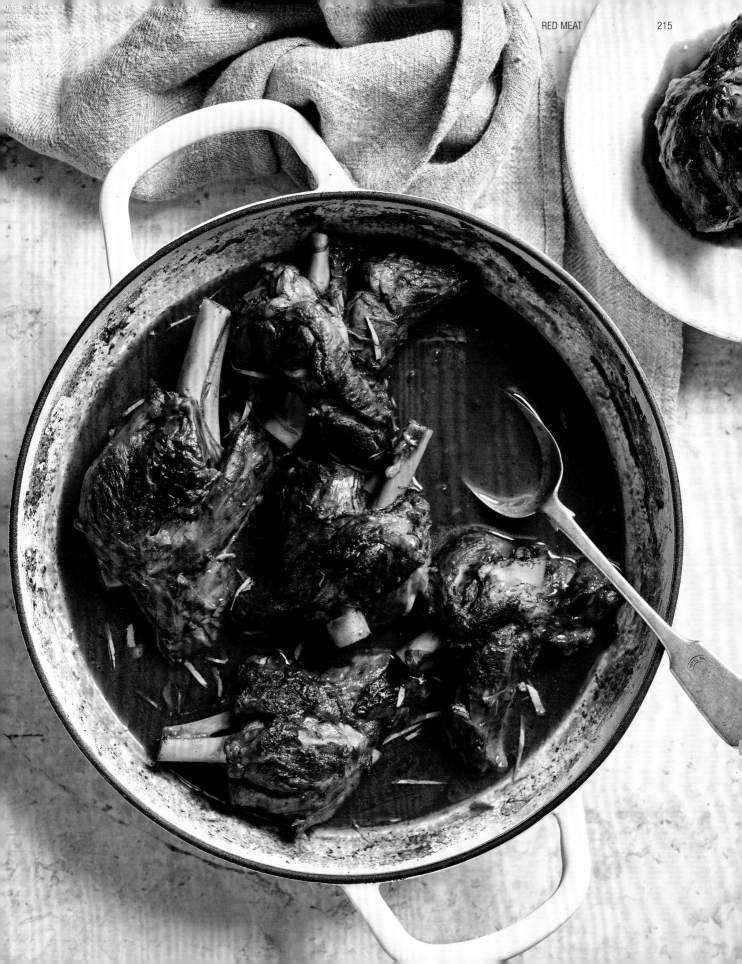

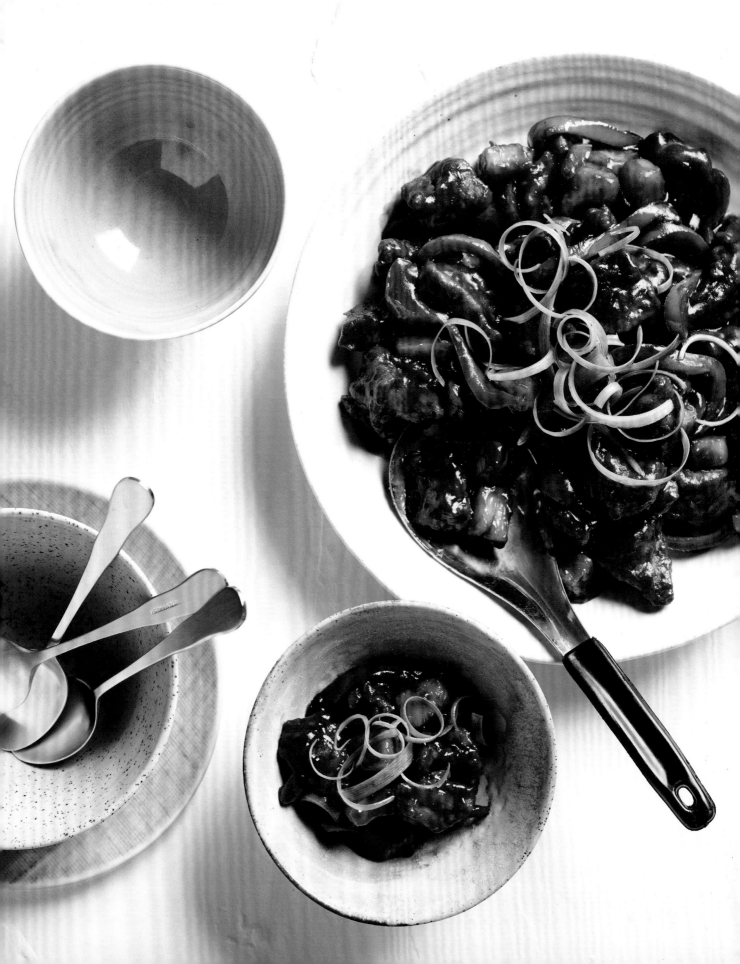

SWEET AND SOUR PORK

SERVES 4

1 tsp five-spice powder

2 tsp light soy sauce

2 tsp Shaoxing wine

1 egg, beaten

500g (1lb) pork neck, cut into 3cm
(1¼ inch) cubes

vegetable oil for deep frying

1 cup gluten-free flour (for dusting)

2–3 long red chillies, deseeded and
finely diced

1 tsp vegetable oil, extra, for
shallow frying

1 tsp garlic-infused olive oil

1 green capsicum (bell pepper),
deseeded and cut into strips

250g (9oz) fresh pineapple, cut into
2cm (¾ inch) chunks

2 tbsp cornflour (cornstarch)

1 tbsp water

½ cup spring onions (scallions) (green
tops only), finely sliced

SAUCE

¾ cup low FODMAP chicken stock

⅓ cup tomato sauce (low
FODMAP ketchup)

1 tbsp caster sugar

1 tbsp white vinegar

2 tsp light soy sauce

2 tsp dark soy sauce

½ tsp sesame oil

Energy 1806kJ/432 Calories, Protein
45.7g, Total Fat 12.1g, Saturated Fat 2.7g,
Carbohydrate 32.1g, Sugars 17.1g, Dietary
fibre 4.3g, Calcium 57.5mg, Iron 3.4mg.

1. To marinate the pork, combine the five-spice, light soy, Shaoxing wine, egg and a pinch of salt in a bowl.

2. Add the pork and mix well. Cover with plastic wrap and refrigerate to marinate for at least 15 minutes or overnight (if marinating overnight, mix in the egg just before cooking).

3. To make the sweet and sour sauce, mix the chicken stock, tomato sauce (low FODMAP ketchup), caster sugar, vinegar, soy sauces and sesame oil in a bowl. Set aside.

4. Combine the flour and pork in a bowl and toss to coat the pork, shaking off any excess flour. Set the pork aside.

5. Pour oil into a wok or large saucepan to a depth of 5cm (2 inches) and heat over high heat until the oil is shimmering. Deep-fry the pork in batches until browned and crisp (3-4 minutes). Remove the pork and drain on a paper towel. Repeat if desired for a crisper texture. Discard the oil when cool.

6. Heat the extra teaspoon of vegetable oil and the garlic-infused olive oil in a clean pan over hight heat. Add the chilli and stir for a few seconds, then add the capsicum and pineapple. Stir-fry for 20 seconds to coat with oil.

7. Add the sweet and sour sauce, bring to the boil and cook until warmed through (30-40 seconds).

8. Combine the cornflour (cornstarch) with the water and stir into boiling sauce to thicken.

9. Add the pork to the sauce and warm through (1-2 minutes). Serve garnished with spring onion(scallion) tops.

SERVING SUGGESTION

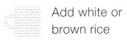
Add white or
brown rice

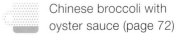
Chinese broccoli with
oyster sauce (page 72)

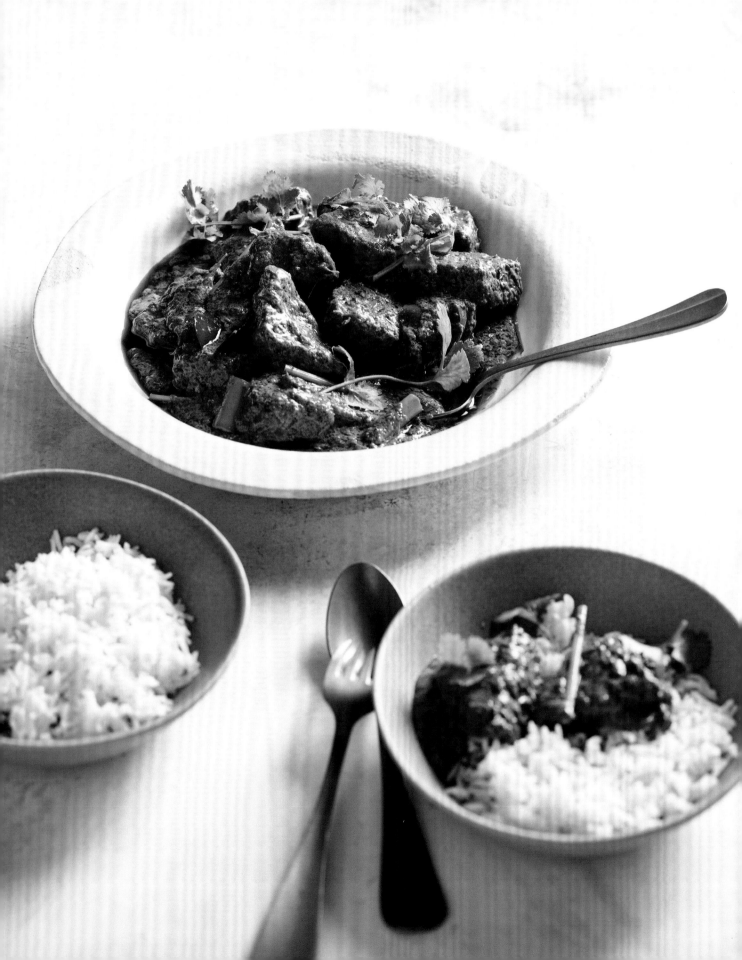

MALAYSIAN BEEF CURRY

SERVES 8

3 cups roughly chopped spring onions
  (scallions) (green tops only)

4 fresh long red chillies, deseeded and
  roughly chopped

2.5cm (1 inch) piece fresh turmeric,
  peeled and roughly chopped

10cm (4 inch) piece fresh ginger,
  peeled and roughly chopped

2.5cm (1 inch) piece galangal, peeled
  and roughly chopped

1 tbsp ground turmeric

30g (1oz) tamarind paste

⅓ cup vegetable oil

2 lemongrass stalks, tough outer leaves
  removed and stalks roughly chopped

4 makrut (kaffir) lime leaves,
  roughly torn

sea salt and pepper to taste

1kg (2lb) beef topside, diced into 4cm
  (1½ inch) pieces

2 cups coconut milk

½ cup coriander (cilantro) leaves

Energy 1523.8kJ/364 Calories, Protein
28.9g, Total Fat 25.4g, Saturated Fat 11.4g,
Carbohydrate 4.8g, Sugars 3.2g, Dietary
fibre 1.7g, Calcium 16.4mg, Iron 3.2mg.

1. Add the spring onion (scallion) tops, chillies, fresh turmeric, ginger, galangal, ground turmeric and tamarind to a food processor bowl. Pulse until a thick paste forms.

2. In a large pan over medium heat, heat the vegetable oil. Add in the chilli paste, lemongrass, lime leaves, sea salt and pepper. Cook for 5 minutes then set aside.

3. In a separate pan over high heat, sear the diced beef for 10 minutes, or until the meat begins to brown. Add the curry paste and stir well to coat the meat.

4. Stir in the coconut milk, cover and cook for 1–1½ hours, or until the meat is tender and the paste has thickened.

5. Scatter the coriander leaves over the curry and serve with cooked rice.

SERVING SUGGESTION

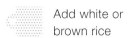
Add white or
brown rice

CHINESE BRAISED BEEF NOODLES

SERVES 4

500g (1lb) beef short ribs, sliced into individual ribs or cut into pieces

500g (1lb) chuck steak or gravy beef, cut into 4cm (1½ inch) pieces

sea salt to taste

1 tbsp vegetable oil

1 tbsp garlic-infused olive oil

30g (1oz) ginger, peeled and finely julienned

½ cup Shaoxing wine

2 star anise, whole

1 tsp cinnamon

1 tsp Chinese five spice

¼ cup light soy sauce

1 tbsp dark soy sauce

1 tbsp tomato paste

2 tbsp brown sugar

2 cups water

400g (14oz) thick rice noodles

1 tsp sesame oil

2 tbsp cornflour (cornstarch)

1 tbsp water

¼ cup spring onions (scallions) (green tops only), roughly chopped

¼ cup coriander (cilantro)

Energy 2645kJ/632 Calories, Protein 52.6g, Total Fat 29.1g, Saturated Fat 8.3g, Carbohydrate 37.8g, Sugars 9.7g, Dietary fibre 2.8g, Calcium 65.9mg, Iron 6.0mg.

1. Preheat the oven to 160°C/320°F. Heat the oil in a large heavy-based saucepan over high heat. Using a paper towel, pat the beef to remove the surface moisture and season with salt.

2. Add the beef to the pan in batches and sear until a brown crust forms. Remove the beef and set aside on a plate.

3. Add the garlic-infused olive oil and ginger to the pan and cook for another 30 seconds. Deglaze the saucepan with the Shaoxing wine, and use a wooden spoon to scrape up the brown beef residue on the bottom of the pan.

4. Return the beef and its juices to the pan. Add the star anise, cinnamon, Chinese five spice, soy sauces, tomato paste, brown sugar and water. Mix well. Bring the mixture to a simmer, cover with a lid and transfer to the oven. Cook for 1½–2 hours or until the beef is tender enough to pierce with a fork.

5. When the beef is almost ready, cook the noodles in boiling water for 5 minutes or until just tender. Drain the noodles and add the sesame oil. Toss the noodles with tongs or chopsticks until the noodles have cooled to room temperature; this will prevent the noodles from sticking together.

6. Remove the star anise from the braise (discard). Remove the beef ribs with a slotted spoon and transfer to a chopping board. Remove the bones and slice the meat.

7. Ladle any excess fat from the top of the sauce (discard). If the sauce is too runny, combine the cornflour with the water and stir the mixture into the sauce.

8. Add the sliced beef back into the sauce and stir over low heat until the sauce has thickened and the beef is heated through.

9. Divide the noodles and beef between serving bowls, top with spring onion (scallion) tops and coriander, and serve.

SERVING SUGGESTION

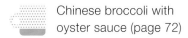
Chinese broccoli with oyster sauce (page 72)

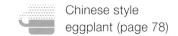
Chinese style eggplant (page 78)

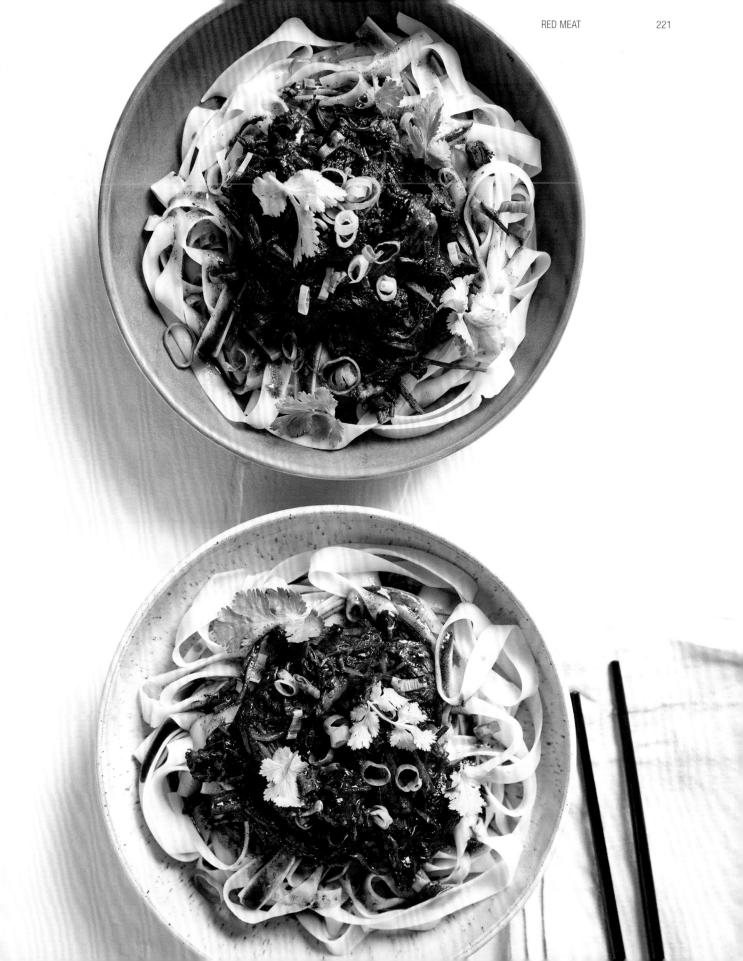

BEEF BURGUNDY

SERVES 6

1kg (2lb) chuck steak (beef brisket),
  cut into 5cm (2 inch) chunks
¼ tsp salt
¼ tsp freshly ground pepper
2 tbsp garlic-infused olive oil
120g (4oz) bacon, chopped
1½ cups spring onions (scallions)
  (green tops only), finely chopped
1 large carrot, chopped
2 cups red wine
2 cups low FODMAP beef stock
1 low FODMAP beef stock (beef
  bouillon) cube
2 tbsp tomato paste
2 tbsp cornflour (cornstarch)
1 tsp fresh thyme
2 tbsp chopped parsley
2 bay leaves
2 tbsp butter
300g (10½oz) oyster mushrooms, cut
  into strips
2 tbsp chopped parsley extra to serve

Energy 2012kJ/481 Calories, Protein
43.1g, Total Fat 23.1g, Saturated Fat 7.4g,
Carbohydrate 7.8g, Sugars 4.8g, Dietary
fibre 3.4g, Calcium 52mg, Iron 5.1mg.

1. Preheat the oven to 160°C/320°F.

2. Cut the meat into large pieces. Pat dry with absorbent paper and rub with salt and ground pepper.

3. Heat the oil in a large heavy-based casserole over medium heat. Add the bacon and fry until cooked through, stirring occasionally. Remove the bacon and set aside.

4. Reduce the heat to low and add the finely chopped spring onion (scallion) tops, and chopped carrots. Cook for 2–3 minutes. Remove from the casserole dish and set aside.

5. Increase the heat to high and brown the meat pieces in four separate batches, adding extra oil if necessary. Repeat until all the meat is browned, then return all the meat to the casserole.

6. Return the bacon, spring onion tops and carrot to the casserole. Sprinkle the cornflour (cornstarch) over the meat and stir well. Cook for 2–3 minutes.

7. Add the wine, beef stock, tomato paste, bouillon cube and fresh herbs (thyme, parsley, bay leaves) and bring to a simmer. Cover the casserole dish with a lid and place in the bottom of the oven. Cook for 2–3 hours or until the meat is very tender.

8. Meanwhile, heat a frypan over medium heat, add the butter, then add the sliced mushrooms. Cook for 5–10 min or until the mushrooms are browned. Set aside.

9. When the meat is cooked, remove the casserole from the oven and gently stir through the cooked mushrooms.

10. Thin the sauce if necessary by adding more stock.

11. Serve sprinkled with the extra parsley.

SERVING SUGGESTION

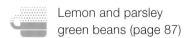
Lemon and parsley
green beans (page 87)

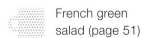
French green
salad (page 51)

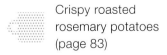
Crispy roasted
rosemary potatoes
(page 83)

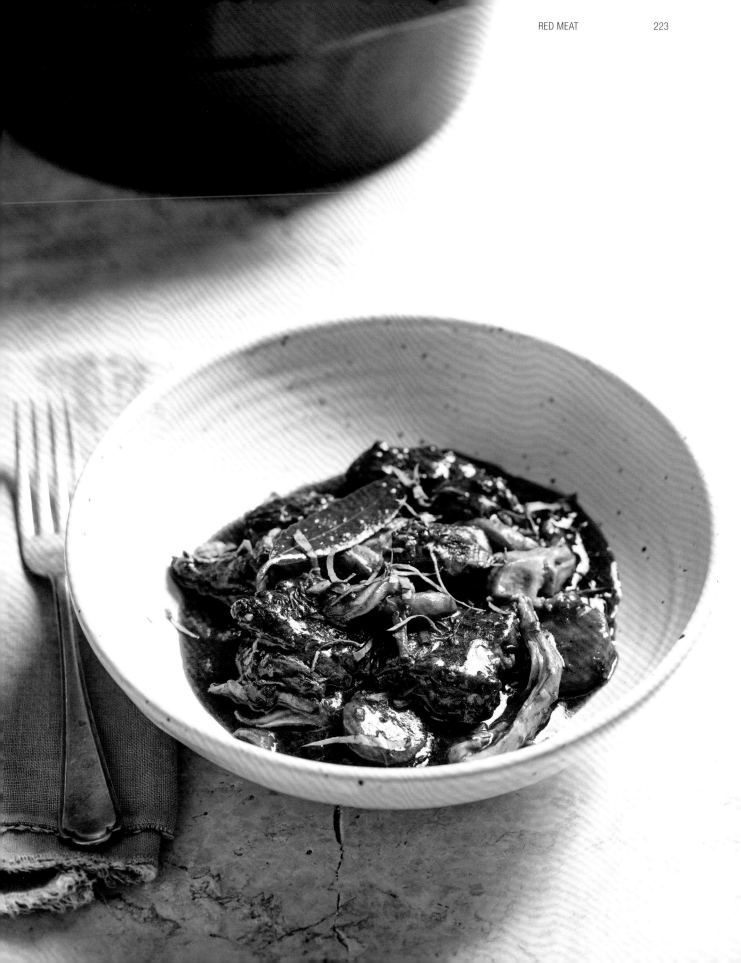

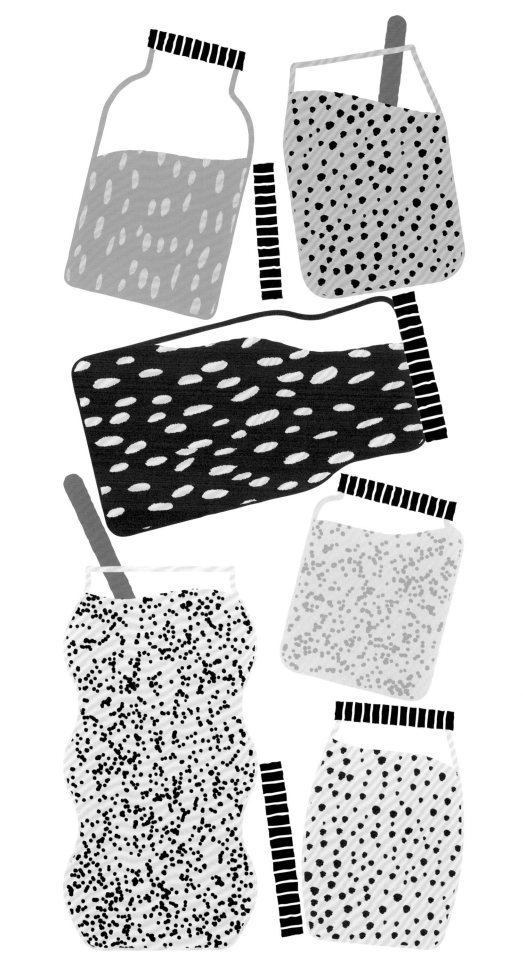

BASICS

CHICKEN STOCK

SERVES 8

1kg (2lb) chicken carcasses or
   chicken bones
300g (10½oz) leek greens,
   roughly chopped
2 carrots, chopped
6 parsley sprigs
2 thyme sprigs
10 peppercorns
3 bay leaves
4L (8½pt) water

1. Place all ingredients in a large, deep saucepan and cover with water. Bring to the boil and then reduce to a simmer, skimming the surface as needed.

2. Simmer uncovered for 4 hours or until the liquid has reduced by half. Let sit for 30 minutes and then strain. Refrigerate in an airtight container for up to 1 week or freeze for later use.

Energy 130kJ/31 Calories, Protein 4.1g,
Total Fat 1.1g, Saturated Fat 0.4g,
Carbohydrate 1.4g, Sugars 1.4g, Dietary
fibre 0g, Calcium 8.1mg, Iron 0.1mg.

VEGETABLE STOCK

SERVES 8

3 tbsp garlic-infused olive oil
300g (10½oz) leek greens,
   roughly chopped
1 swede, peeled and roughly chopped
2 carrots, roughly chopped
3½L (7½pt) water
10 parsley sprigs
4 thyme sprigs
10 peppercorns, whole
3 bay leaves
salt to taste

1. Heat the oil in a large saucepan over medium heat. Add the leek greens, swede and carrot and cook for 5 minutes.

2. Add the water, tomato, parsley, thyme, peppercorns and bay leaves and bring to the boil. Reduce heat to low and simmer for 2 hours uncovered, skimming as necessary. Cover partly with a lid and simmer for another 1½–2 hours.

3. Set aside for 30 minutes and then carefully strain the stock through a sieve. Refrigerate in an airtight container for up to 1 week or freeze for later use.

Energy 129k/31 CaloriesJ, Protein 3.1g,
Total Fat 1.1g, Saturated Fat 0.4g,
Carbohydrate 2.3g, Sugars 2.3g, Dietary
fibre 0g, Calcium 8.1mg, Iron 0.1mg.

BEEF STOCK

SERVES 8

1kg (2lb) beef bones

5–6L (11-12pt) water

1 cup spring onions (scallions) (green
   tops only), finely chopped

1 medium-sized carrot, chopped

3–4 parsley sprigs

1 strip lemon zest

1 bay leaf

2 thyme sprigs

1 tsp black peppercorns

1 tsp coriander seeds

Energy 150kJ/36 Calories, Protein 4.2g,
Total Fat 1.3g, Saturated Fat 0.4g,
Carbohydrate 2.0g, Sugars 1.5g, Dietary
fibre 0g, Calcium 8.1mg, Iron 0.1mg.

1. Preheat the oven to 200°C/400°F. Roast the beef bones for
   45–60 minutes or until brown.

2. Transfer the bones to a large, deep stock pot. Add the water
   (make sure the bones are covered) and simmer on medium-low
   heat for 2–3 minutes.

3. Add the spring onion (scallion) tops, carrot, parsley, lemon zest,
   bay leaf, thyme, black peppercorns and coriander seeds to
   the pot.

4. Gently simmer the stock for 4–6 hours over low heat.

5. Strain the stock through a fine sieve. Refrigerate until chilled,
   then remove and discard any fat that sets on the top.
   Refrigerate in an airtight container for up to 3 days, or freeze
   for up to 6 months.

FRENCH DRESSING

SERVES 5
2 tbsp white wine vinegar
¼ tsp sea salt
2 tsp Dijon mustard
⅓ cup olive oil

Energy 563kJ/135 Calories, Protein 0.2g,
Total Fat 15.0g, Saturated Fat 2.3g,
Carbohydrate 0.1g, Sugars 0.1g, Dietary
fibre 0.1g, Calcium 2.1mg, Iron 0.0mg.

1. Add the vinegar, salt, mustard and oil to a jar with a tight fitting lid and shake vigorously. The dressing can be stored in the fridge for 3–4 weeks.

'GARLIC' AIOLI

SERVES 14
1 large egg yolk
¼ tsp white sugar
¼ tsp sea salt flakes
1 tbsp lemon juice
¾ cup olive oil
¼ cup garlic-infused olive oil
1½ tbsp water, or as required
¼ tsp freshly ground black pepper

Energy 624.4kJ/149 Calories, Protein 0.2g,
Total Fat 16.7g, Saturated Fat 2.6g,
Carbohydrate 0.1g, Sugars 0.1g, Dietary
fibre 0g, Calcium 1.4mg, Iron 0.1mg.

1. Place the egg yolks, sugar, salt and lemon juice in a food processor bowl.

2. Blitz in the food processor until well combined, then gradually add the oils in a thin, steady stream. As the aioli thickens, add a little of the water. Continue to blitz until all the oil is incorporated. Adjust the consistency to your taste by adding extra water.

3. Season with pepper and additional salt if desired. Store in an airtight container in the fridge for up to 2 weeks.

MAYONNAISE

SERVES 10

1 egg yolk

¼ tsp white sugar

¼ tsp salt

¼ tsp pepper

1 tbsp lemon juice

1 cup canola oil

1 tbsp water, or as required

Energy 875kJ/209 Calories, Protein 0.3g,
Total Fat 23.5g, Saturated Fat 1.8g,
Carbohydrate 0.2g, Sugars 0.2g, Dietary
fibre 0g, Calcium 2.2mg, Iron 0.1mg.

1. Place the egg yolks, sugar, salt, pepper and lemon juice into a food processor.

2. Blitz in the food processor until well combined, then gradually add the oil in a thin, steady stream. As the mayonnaise thickens, add a little of the water. Continue to blitz until all the oil is incorporated. Adjust the consistency to your taste by adding extra water.

3. Store in an airtight container in the fridge for up to 2 weeks.

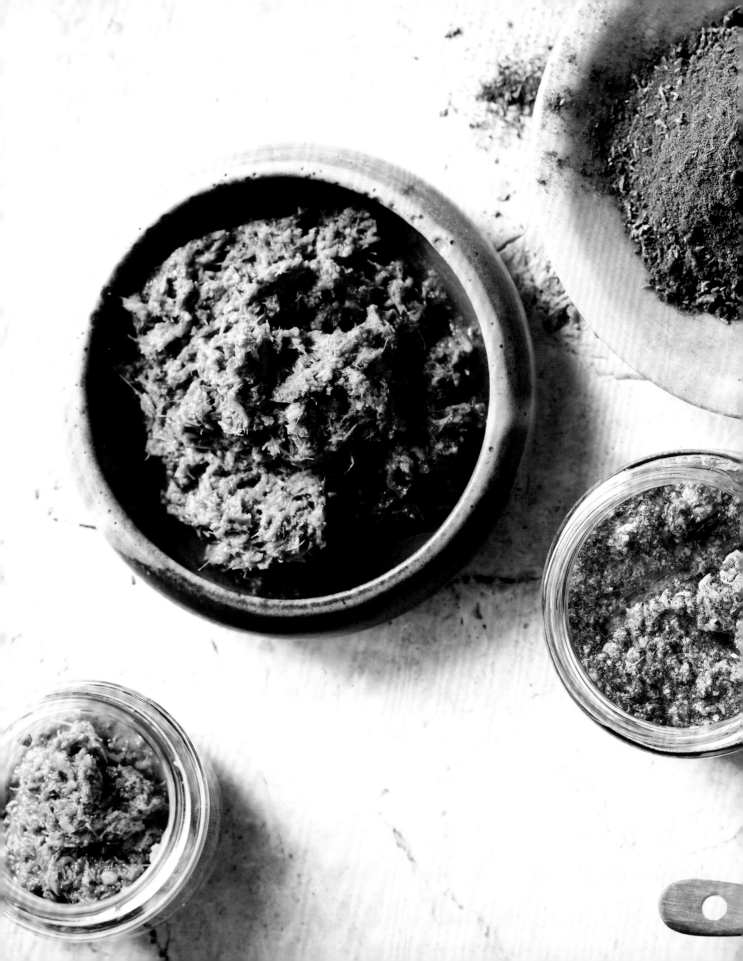

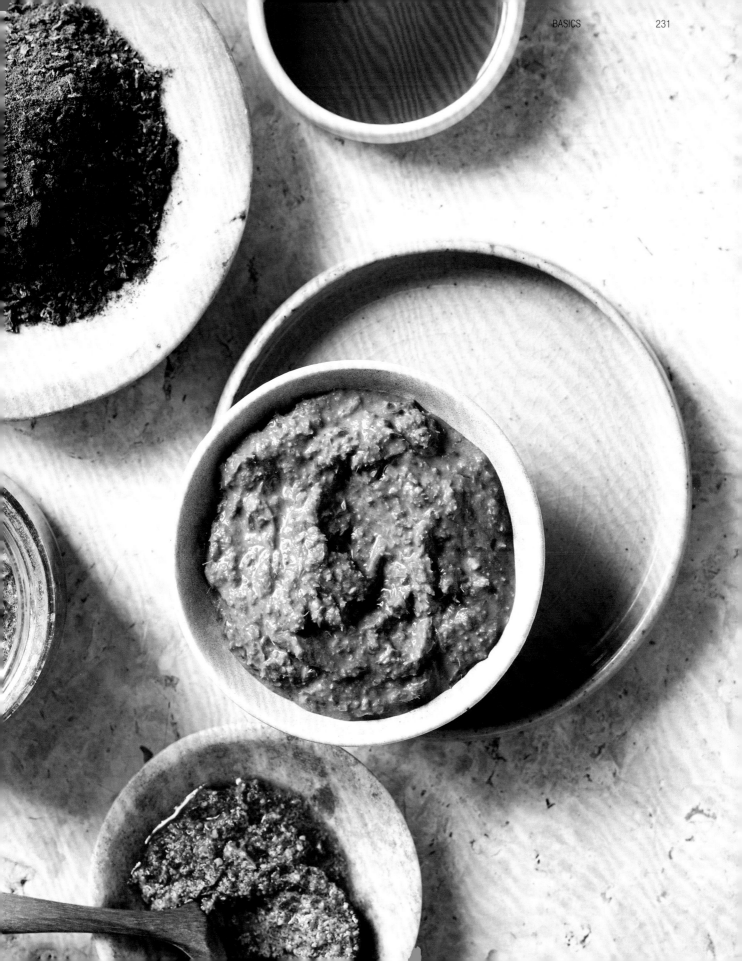

LACTOSE-FREE NATURAL GREEK YOGHURT

SERVES 4

1 Lacteeze tablet

200g (7oz) natural Greek yoghurt

Energy 200kJ/48 Calories, Protein 2.0g, Total Fat 3.2g, Saturated Fat 3.2g, Carbohydrate 2.3g, Sugars 2.3g, Dietary fibre 0g, Calcium 58mg, Iron 0.0mg.

1. Grind the Lacteeze tablet in a bowl with the back of a spoon.

2. Add the yoghurt and mix well.

3. Place the yoghurt in a jar with a well-fitting lid and set aside in the fridge overnight.

4. Use the lactose-free yoghurt within 2–3 days.

PESTO

SERVES 4

⅓ cup pine nuts

2 cups basil leaves, packed

¼ cup grated parmesan

1 tbsp lemon juice

½ cup garlic-infused olive oil

salt and pepper to taste

Energy 1676kJ/401 Calories, Protein 5.3g, Total Fat 41.7g, Saturated Fat 6.5g, Carbohydrate 1.3g, Sugars 0.5g, Dietary fibre 2.2g, Calcium 150.4mg, Iron 1.2mg.

1. In a small frypan, toast the pine nuts over medium heat for approximately 3 minutes, stirring frequently to ensure the nuts don't burn. Set aside in a bowl to cool.

2. To make the pesto, add the pine nuts, basil leaves, parmesan and lemon juice to a food processor. Blitz until finely chopped. Slowly pour in the garlic-infused olive oil while the processor is running and blitz until combined. Season with salt and pepper.

3. Store the pesto in an airtight container in the refrigerator for up to a week.

INDIAN CORIANDER AND MINT RAITA

SERVES 5

1 tsp cumin seeds

1 tsp black mustard seeds

200g (7oz) lactose-free natural Greek
yoghurt (see page 232)

⅓ cup fresh mint leaves, chopped

⅓ cup coriander (cilantro) leaves,
chopped

1 fresh green chilli, chopped

1½ tbsp lime juice

¼ tsp salt, or to taste

Energy 226kJ/54 Calories, Protein 2.9g,
Total Fat 1.7g, Saturated Fat 1.1g,
Carbohydrate 6.2g, Sugars 5.3g, Dietary
fibre 0.9g, Calcium 89.6mg, Iron 0.7mg.

1. Heat a heavy-based non-stick frypan over medium heat and roast the cumin seeds and mustard seeds until aromatic.

2. Cool the roasted seeds and grind or pound them to a fine powder in a small food processor or mortar and pestle.

3. Place the ground, roasted seeds into a small food processor. Add the lactose-free yoghurt, mint leaves, coriander leaves and green chilli and blend until the herbs are finely chopped and the mixture is smooth.

4. Add the pinch of salt and lime juice and mix well. Adjust the seasoning to taste.

5. Refrigerate until ready to serve.

TACO SEASONING

SERVES 30

½ cup ground cumin

⅓ cup smoked paprika

2 tbsp chilli powder

2 tbsp dried oregano

1 tbsp black pepper

Energy 72.7kJ/17 Calories, Protein 0.7g,
Total Fat 0.8g, Saturated Fat 0.1g,
Carbohydrate 1.3g, Sugars 0.3g, Dietary
fibre 1.2g, Calcium 35.9mg, Iron 2.0mg.

1. Combine all ingredients in a jar or zip lock bag. Shake well until combined. Store in the pantry in an airtight container.

2. Use 1½ tbsp of the taco seasoning per 500g of protein. Season with salt to taste.

THAI GREEN CURRY PASTE

SERVES 6

½ tsp ground coriander

1 tsp ground cumin

½ tsp ground pepper

100g (3½oz) fresh green chillies,
   stems and most seeds removed

1½ lemongrass stalks,
   roughly chopped

2cm (¾ inch) piece galangal,
   roughly chopped

20g (¾oz) spring onions (scallions)
   (green tops only)

1 tsp ground turmeric

2 tbsp coriander, including roots and
   stems, roughly chopped

½ tsp sea salt

⅓ cup juice and zest of 1 lime

2 tbsp garlic-infused olive oil

1 tbsp brown sugar

Energy 329kJ/79 Calories, Protein 0.8g,
Total Fat 6.4g, Saturated Fat 1.0g,
Carbohydrate 3.0g, Sugars 2.6g, Dietary
fibre 3g, Calcium 16.0mg, Iron 1.0mg.

1. Add all the ingredients to a food processor and pulse on high until a paste forms. Scrape down the sides as necessary.

2. Store the paste in an airtight container in the refrigerator for up to a week, or freeze for later use.

THAI RED CURRY PASTE

SERVES 6

40g (1½oz) dried chillies,
   seeds discarded
1 lemongrass stalk, sliced
1 tbsp grated galangal
1 tbsp coriander roots
2 tsp shrimp paste
½ tsp ground coriander
½ tsp ground cumin
1 tsp lime zest
¼ cup water
1 tbsp garlic-infused oil

Energy 438kJ/105 Calories, Protein 2.0g,
Total Fat 9.6g, Saturated Fat 1.5g,
Carbohydrate 1.6g, Sugars 0.5g, Dietary
fibre 2.5g, Calcium 104.5mg, Iron 2.4mg.

1. Chop dried chillies into 1cm (½ inch) pieces. Add to a bowl of hot water and soak for 20 minutes.

2. Drain the chillies and add to a blender.

3. Add all the other ingredients to the blender and blitz on high until smooth.

4. Store the paste in an airtight container in the refrigerator for up to a week, or freeze for later use.

SICHUAN CHILLI OIL

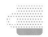

SERVES 10

1 cup oil (vegetable or canola)
4 star anise, whole
1 cinnamon stick
2 tbsp Sichuan peppercorns
1½ tbsp chilli powder
2 tbsp garlic-infused olive oil
1 tsp sea salt

Energy 995kJ/238 Calories, Protein 0.0g,
Total Fat 26.8g, Saturated Fat 3.0g,
Carbohydrate 0.1g, Sugars 0.0g, Dietary
fibre 0.3g, Calcium 4.1mg, Iron 0.1mg.

1. Place the oil (vegetable or canola) in a saucepan over low heat.

2. In a separate pan over medium-high heat, toast the star anise, cinnamon stick and Sichuan peppercorns until the ingredients start to smoke.

3. Add the cooked spices to the warm oil.

4. Increase the heat to medium and cook the spices in the oil for 4–5 minutes. The spices should begin to gently sizzle. Remove the saucepan from the heat and cool for 5 minutes.

5. Strain the spiced oil into a bowl (discard the spices). Stir in the remaining ingredients. Store in an airtight jar.

TONKATSU SAUCE

SERVES 10

½ cup tomato sauce (low
  FODMAP ketchup)
2 tbsp soy sauce
1 tbsp brown sugar
1 tbsp mirin
1½ tsp Worcestershire sauce
1 tsp grated ginger

Energy 120kJ/29 Calories, Protein 0.5g,
Total Fat 0.0g, Saturated Fat 0.0g,
Carbohydrate 6.2g, Sugars 6.0g, Dietary
fibre 0.2g, Calcium 6.1mg, Iron 0.2mg.

1. Whisk all ingredients together in a bowl.

2. Set aside for 30 minutes before serving to allow the flavours to
    blend.

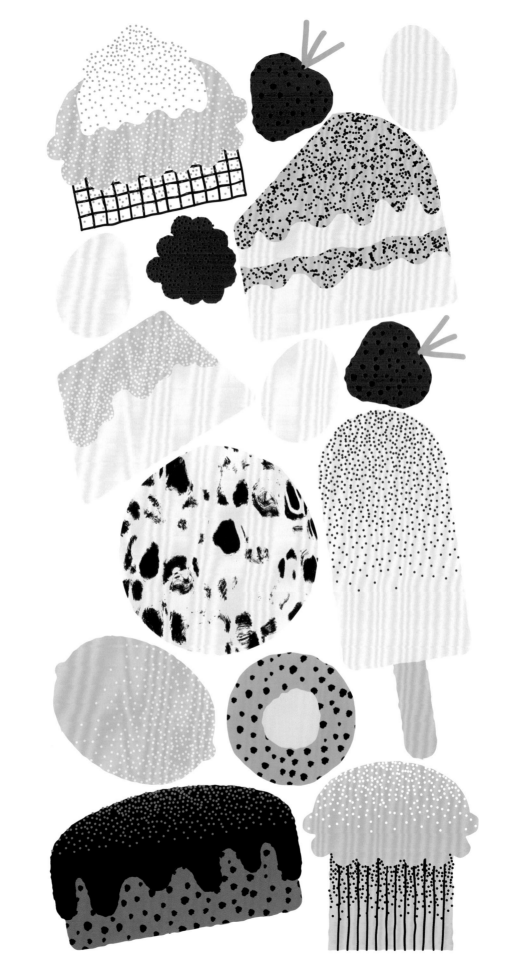

SWEETS

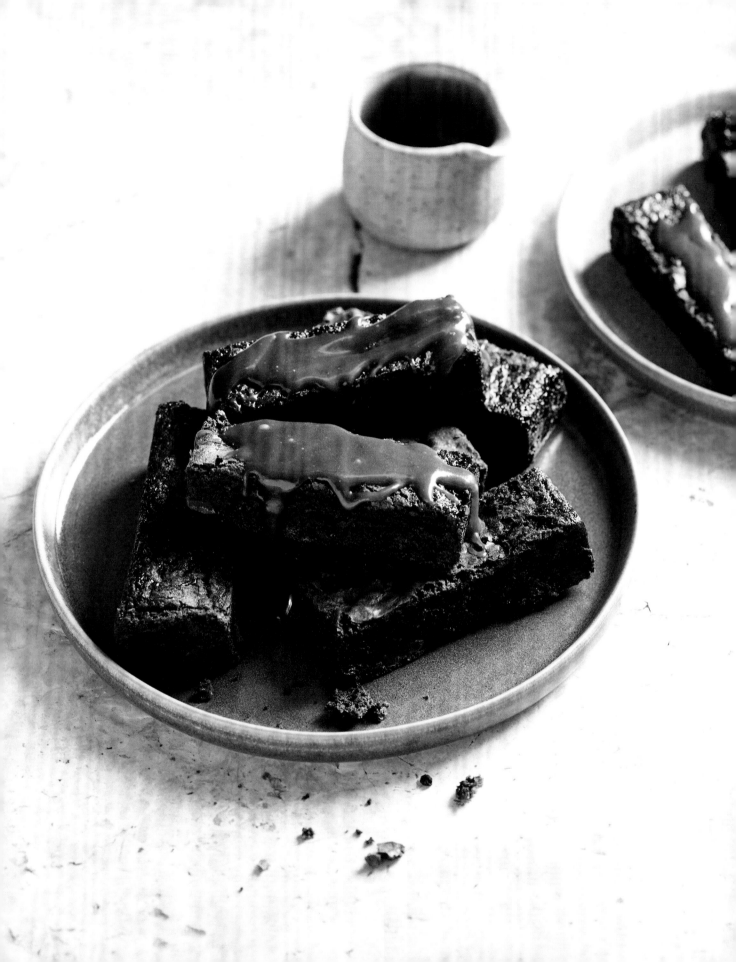

FUDGY BROWNIES WITH MISO CARAMEL

SERVES 12

MISO SAUCE
2 tbsp white miso paste
2 tbsp warm water
¾ cup (170g/6oz) castor sugar
¼ cup water, extra
⅓ cup (80ml/2½ fl oz)
   thickened cream

BROWNIE MIXTURE
170g (6oz) unsalted butter, melted
1 cup (225g/8oz) castor sugar
½ cup (75g/2½oz) brown sugar
1 tsp vanilla essence (extract)
3 eggs
½ cup cocoa powder
½ cup gluten-free flour
75g (2½oz) dark chocolate chips

Energy 1573kJ/376 Calories, Protein 3.9g,
Total Fat 19.0g, Saturated Fat 11.7g,
Carbohydrate 46.4g, Sugars 39.9g, Dietary
fibre 1.5g, Calcium 38.7mg, Iron 2.0mg.

1. Preheat the oven to 180°C/350°F.

2. Line a 20cm (8 inch) square baking tin with baking paper. Ensure the baking paper overhangs the sides of the tin.

3. To make the miso caramel, whisk together the miso paste and 2 tbsp warm water in a small bowl until smooth. Set aside.

4. In a saucepan, heat sugar and ¼ cup water over medium-high heat, stirring, until sugar dissolves. Discontinue stirring and bring to the boil. Boil until the sugar turns golden brown.

5. Remove the sugar from the heat and whisk in the cream (be careful, the mixture will bubble and spit). Stir in the miso mixture and set aside.

6. For the brownie mixture, add the melted butter, sugars and vanilla essence to a mixing bowl and whisk to combine.

7. Add the eggs one at a time and combine well. Sift in the cocoa powder and flour and stir until just combined. Fold in the chocolate chips.

8. Spread half the brownie batter into the prepared tin, then drizzle three-quarters of the miso caramel evenly over the top. Finish by spreading the remaining brownie batter over the caramel. Smooth the surface with a spatula.

9. Bake the brownies for 30–35 minutes or until just cooked through.

10. Once cooked, allow all the brownies to cool completely in the tin, then cut into bars.

11. Reheat the remaining miso caramel and serve with the brownies.

LEMON POPPYSEED MUFFINS

SERVES 12

2 cups (300g/10½oz) gluten-free flour

1 tbsp poppy seeds

2 tsp baking powder

¼ tsp baking soda

½ tsp sea salt

⅔ cup (165g/6oz) white sugar

1 lemon, zested and juiced

2 eggs

1 tsp vanilla essence (extract)

⅓ cup vegetable oil (77ml/2¾fl oz)

½ cup unsweetened almond milk

GLAZE

½ cup (60g/2oz) icing sugar

2 tsp lemon juice

half a lemon, zested

Energy 958kJ/289 Calories, Protein 2.3g, Total Fat 8.1g, Saturated Fat 1.0g, Carbohydrate 37.3g, Sugars 18.0g, Dietary fibre 0.5g, Calcium 31.1mg, Iron 0.5mg.

1. Preheat the oven to 200°C/400°F. Line a muffin tray with 12 paper cases.

2. In a large bowl, combine the gluten-free flour, poppy seeds, baking powder, baking soda, salt, sugar and lemon zest. Whisk together and set aside.

3. In a separate medium-sized bowl, beat together the eggs, vanilla extract, lemon juice, oil, and almond milk until well combined.

4. Pour the egg mixture into the flour mixture and whisk until just combined. Distribute the muffin batter evenly among the muffin cases until they are almost full.

5. Bake for approximately 15 minutes, taking care not to over-bake. Remove the muffins from the tray and leave to cool completely on a wire rack.

6. Meanwhile, to make the glaze, whisk together all the glaze ingredients in a small bowl. Spoon the glaze over the muffins and serve.

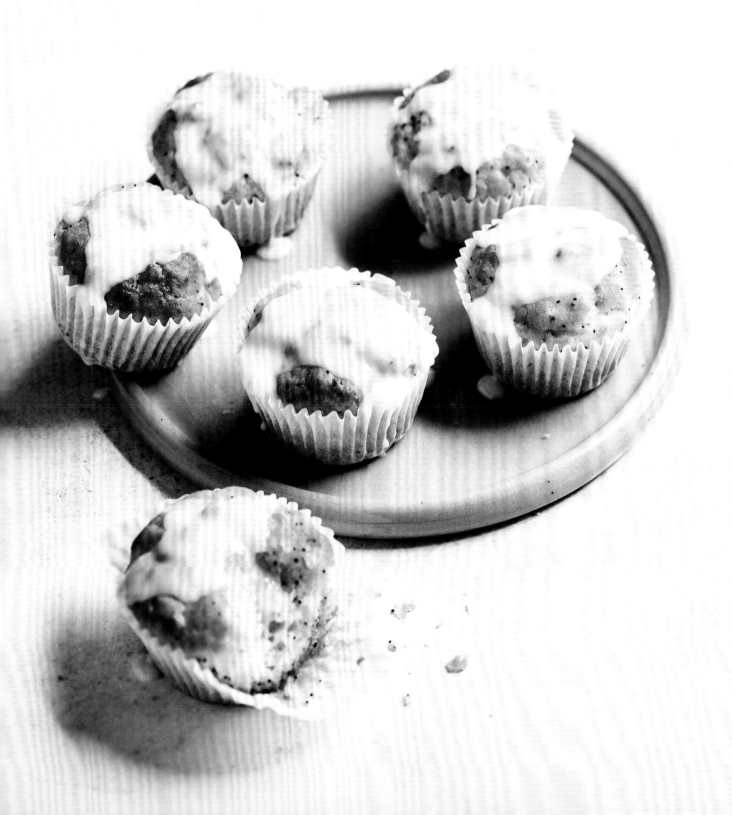

TAHINI CHOCOLATE CHIP COOKIES

SERVES 15

100g (3½oz) unsalted butter
150g (5½oz) tahini
¾ cup (150g/5½oz) sugar
1 egg
1 tsp vanilla essence (extract)
1½ cups (225g/8oz) gluten-free flour
½ tsp baking soda
½ tsp baking powder
1 tsp salt
200g (7oz) dark or milk
   chocolate chips

Energy 1190kJ/284 Calories, Protein
3.8g, Total Fat 17.7g, Saturated Fat 7.9g,
Carbohydrate 27.6g, Sugars 13.9g, Dietary
fibre 1.7g, Calcium 46.2mg, Iron 1.3mg.

1. Preheat the oven to 180°C/350°F and line a baking tray with baking paper.

2. In a medium-sized mixing bowl, use an electric mixer to cream the butter, tahini and sugar for 5 minutes on medium speed. The mixture should be light and creamy.

3. Add the egg and vanilla. Mix for an additional 2 minutes.

4. Sift the flour, baking soda, baking powder and salt into the bowl. Use a spoon or a spatula to mix all ingredients until well combined to form a dough.

5. Stir in most of the chocolate chips, reserving about ¼ cup for decorating.

6. Spoon or roll the dough into 15 balls and placed on the baking tray 5cm (2 inches) apart. Press down slightly.

7. Bake for approximately 15 minutes or until golden brown. Cool for 10-15 minutes, then serve warm or at room temperature.

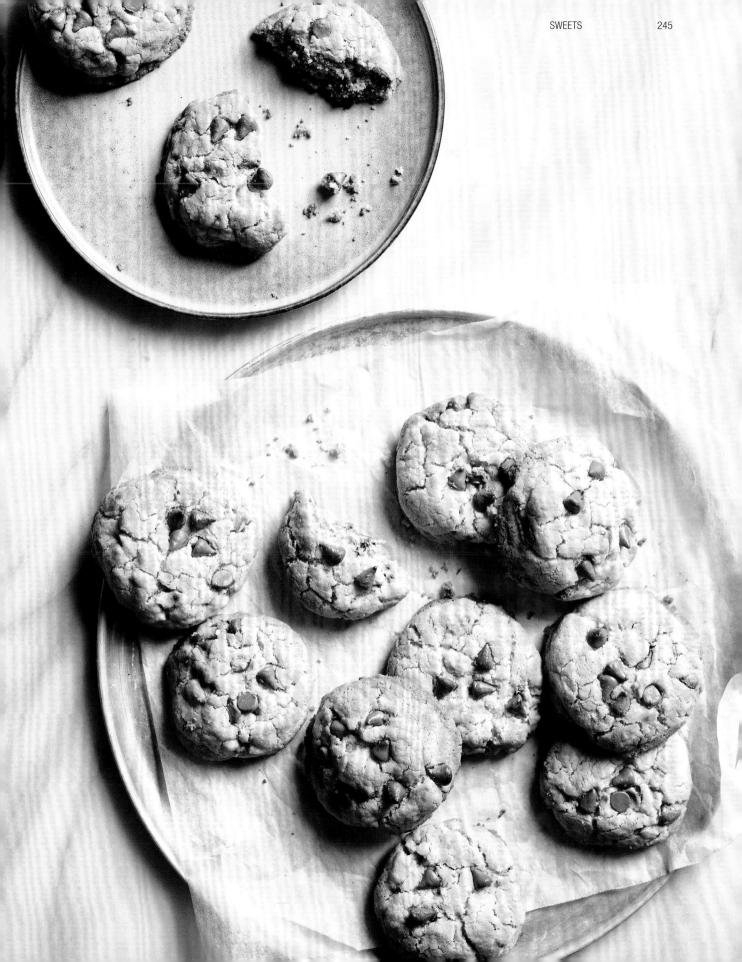

PEANUT BUTTER AND HEMP SEED PROTEIN BALLS

MAKES 9

½ cup (120g/4oz) peanut butter

2 tbsp maple syrup

1 tsp vanilla essence (extract)

⅓ cup hemp seeds

1½ tbsp oat bran

2 tbsp linseeds

¼ cup dark chocolate chips

Energy 729kJ/174 Calories, Protein 5.7g, Total Fat 12.5g, Saturated Fat 2.7g, Carbohydrate 9.0g, Sugars 6.2g, Dietary fibre 2.1g, Calcium 27.5mg, Iron 1.1mg.

1. In a mixing bowl or food processor, thoroughly combine all the ingredients. The mixture should hold together when squeezed into a ball.

2. Using your hands, roll the mixture into 9 balls.

3. Store in the fridge in a sealed container for up to 2 weeks, or wrap individually and freeze for up to 3 months.

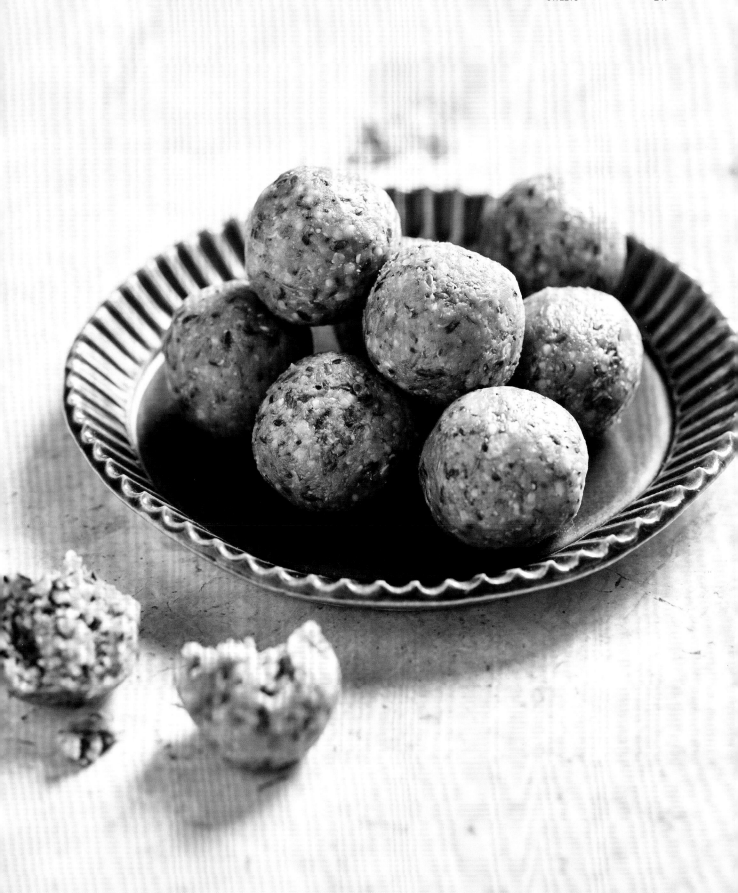

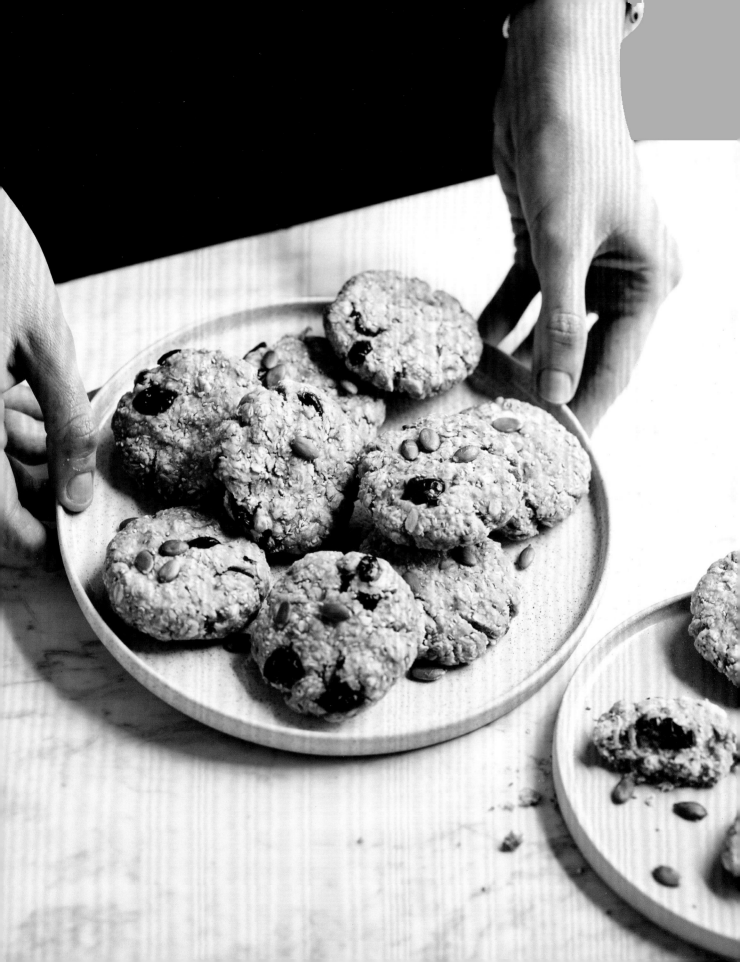

OAT AND SEED BISCUITS

SERVES 12

1½ ripe bananas

2 cups (190g/6½oz) rolled oats

½ cup (75g/2½oz) gluten-free flour

1 tsp cinnamon

2 tbsp chia seeds

2 tbsp dried cranberries,
   roughly chopped

½ tsp baking powder

¼ cup maple syrup

½ cup (120g/4oz) peanut butter

1 tsp vanilla essence (extract)

2 tbsp pepitas

Energy 839kJ/201 Calories, Protein 5.7g,
Total Fat 8.7g, Saturated Fat 1.5g,
Carbohydrate 23.3g, Sugars 8.5g, Dietary
fibre 3.6g, Calcium 39.6mg, Iron 1.3mg.

1. Preheat the oven to 200°C/400°F. Line a baking tray with baking paper.

2. Mash the bananas in a small bowl. Set aside.

3. In a large bowl, mix the rolled oats, gluten-free flour, cinnamon, dried cranberries, chia seeds and baking powder.

4. Stir in the banana, maple syrup, peanut butter and vanilla essence until well combined.

5. Using your hands, roll the mixture into 12 balls. Place them on the tray and press to flatten slightly. Press the pepitas into the biscuits to decorate.

6. Bake for 12–15 minutes or until light golden and cooked through. Transfer to a wire rack to cool. Store in an airtight container for up to 1 week.

BAKLAVA

MAKES 25
10 sheets filo pastry
150ml (5fl oz) extra virgin olive oil
250g (9oz) walnuts
1 tsp cinnamon

SYRUP
1 cup (225g/8oz) castor sugar
¾ cup water
¼ cup pure maple syrup
½ tsp rosewater

Energy 768kJ/184 Calories, Protein 2.2g,
Total Fat 12.7g, Saturated Fat 1.3g,
Carbohydrate 15.4g, Sugars 10.8g, Dietary
fibre 0.9g, Calcium 14.8mg, Iron 0.3mg.

1. Preheat the oven to 200°C/400°F. Line a 28cm x 20cm x 2.5cm (11 inches x 8 inches x 1 inch) tray with baking paper.

2. Pulse the walnuts and cinnamon in a food processor until crushed. In a medium-sized bowl, combine the crushed walnuts with the cinnamon.

3. Brush one sheet of filo pastry with olive oil. Place a second sheet on top so it sticks to the first. Spread a fifth of the walnut mixture in a straight line across the longest edge of the 2 sheets, leaving a margin of approximately 1cm (½ inch) on each end.

4. Fold the short ends of the pastry over the nuts and brush lightly with olive oil. Roll up the pastry into a long roll to enclose the nuts. Place on the oven tray, seam side down. Repeat the process to form 5 rolls, placing them so they touch each other on the tray.

5. Slice the rolls diagonally into 5cm (2 inch) sections. Pour the remaining oil evenly over the rolls. Place the baklava in the oven and bake for 20–25 minutes or until golden brown. Set aside to cool.

6. To make the syrup, combine the sugar, water, maple syrup and rosewater in a saucepan. Bring to the boil over high heat, stirring continuously to dissolve the sugar. Reduce the heat to medium and simmer for 5 minutes or until the syrup begins to thicken.

7. Pour the hot syrup over the cold pastries and set aside to cool completely in the baking tray. Serve or transfer to an airtight container. Baklava will keep refrigerated for up to 2 weeks.

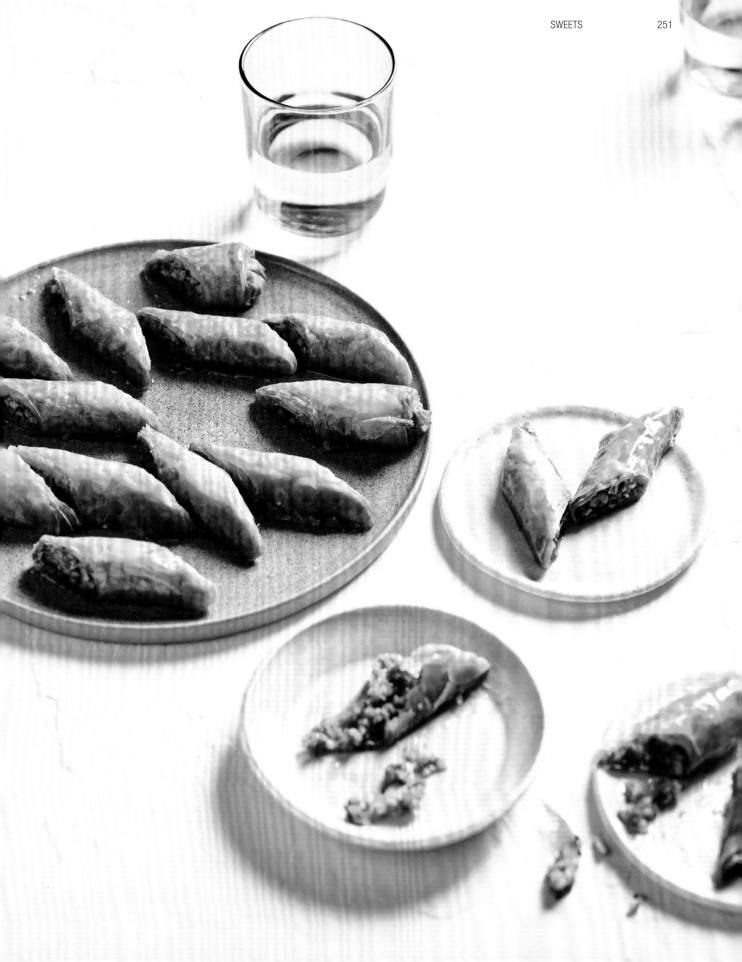

CRÈME CARAMEL

SERVES 6

CARAMEL

1 cup (225g/8oz) castor sugar

½ cup water

CUSTARD

2 whole eggs

2 egg yolks

2 tbsp castor sugar

350ml (12fl oz) lactose-free milk

Energy 960kJ/229 Calories, Protein 4.8g,
Total Fat 4.9g, Saturated Fat 2.1g,
Carbohydrate 43.5g, sugars 43.4g, Dietary
fibre 0.0g, Calcium 79.8mg, Iron 0.5mg.

1. To make the caramel, add the castor sugar and water to a small saucepan. Stir over medium heat until the sugar dissolves.

2. Bring the caramel mixture to the boil without stirring. Using a pastry brush dipped in water, brush the sides of the saucepan to remove sugar crystals.

3. Boil without stirring until the mixture turns light golden. Take care not to burn the caramel as the colour change can occur quickly.

4. Remove the saucepan from the heat and divide the caramel between six ½-cup ovenproof moulds. Rotate the moulds to coat both the bottom and sides with the caramel. Set aside.

5. Preheat the oven to 160°C/320°F.

6. To make the custard, beat together the whole eggs, egg yolks and sugar in a large bowl until well combined.

7. Gently stir in the lactose-free milk and combine well. Strain the mixture through a strainer and into a jug.

8. Divide the custard mixture evenly between the caramel-coated moulds.

9. Place the moulds into a large baking dish and pour hot water into the dish to come halfway up the sides of the moulds.

10. Bake for 25 minutes or until the custard is set.

11. Cool the custard in the fridge overnight.

12. To serve, place a plate over each mould, invert carefully, and shake gently to dislodge the custard onto the plate.

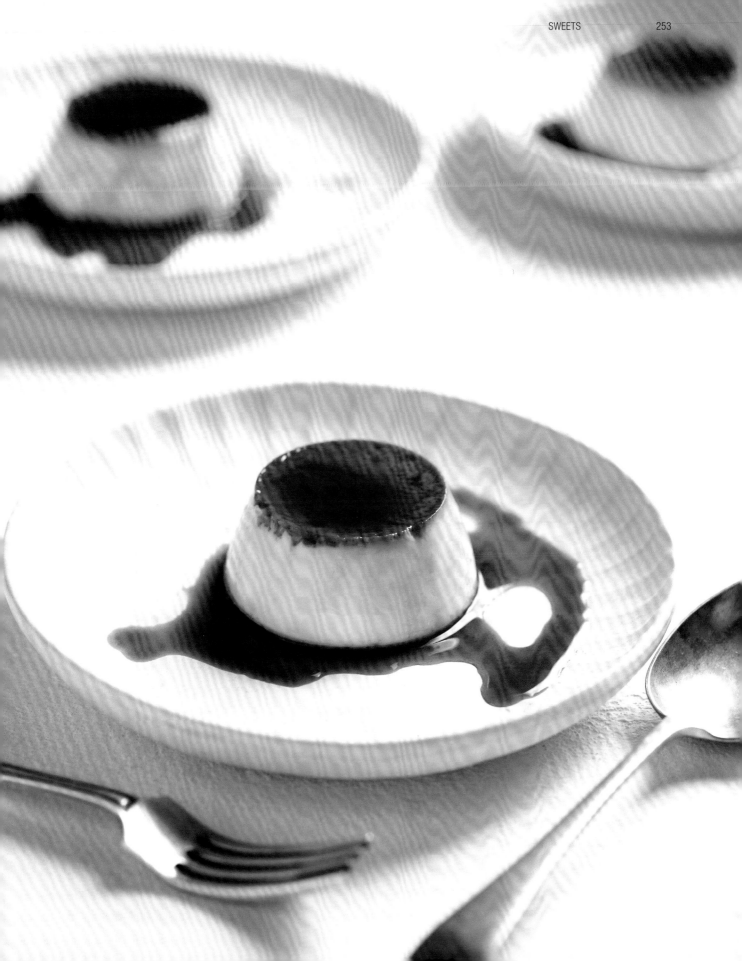

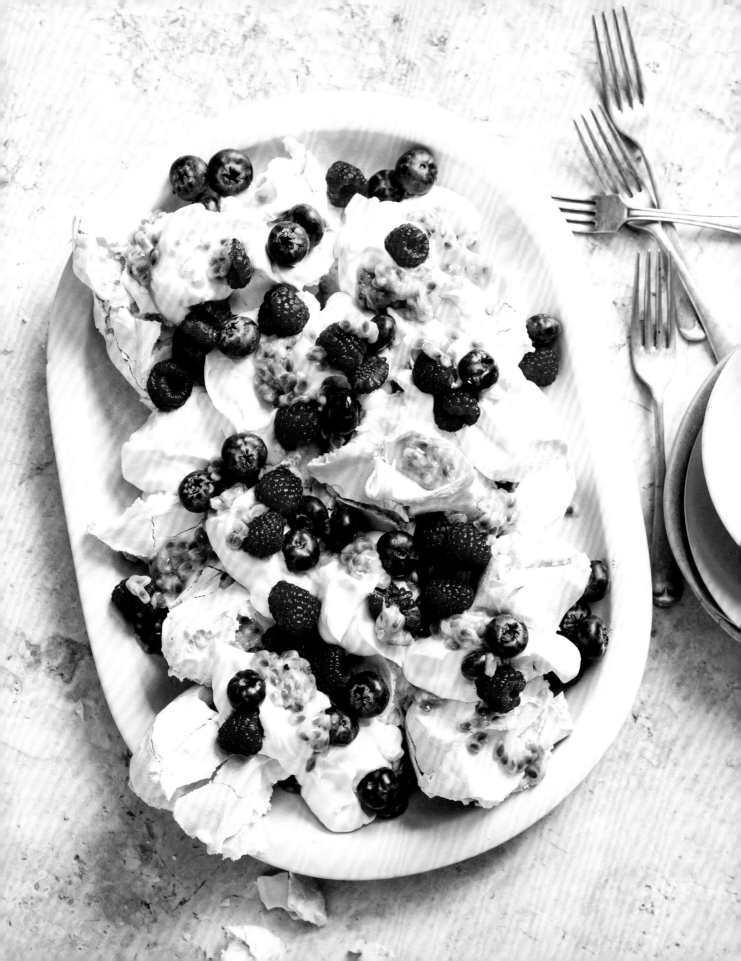

PASSIONFRUIT AND BERRY PAVLOVA CRUNCH

SERVES 6

PAVLOVA
4 egg whites
pinch of salt
1 cup (225g/8oz) castor sugar
½ tsp vanilla essence (extract)
1 tsp white vinegar
2 tsp cornflour (cornstarch)

MIXED FRUIT
125g (4½oz) fresh blueberries
100g (3½oz) fresh passionfruit pulp
125g (4½oz) raspberries (fresh
   or frozen)

CREAM
300ml (10fl oz) lactose-free cream

Energy 1529kJ/366 Calories, Protein 5.1g,
Total Fat 18.7g, Saturated Fat 12.0g,
Carbohydrate 43.9g, sugars 43.2g, Dietary
fibre 4.2g, Calcium 42.1mg, Iron 0.3mg.

1. Preheat the oven to 130°C/270°F and line an oven tray with baking paper.

2. Beat the egg whites and salt with electric beaters until soft peaks form. Gradually add the castor sugar, beating continuously. Add the vinegar and vanilla and keep beating until stiff peaks form.

3. Sift the cornflour (cornstarch) and fold it into the meringue mixture.

4. Spread out onto the oven tray and place on the bottom shelf of your oven. Cook for 1 hour and 30 minutes.

5. Cool completely on the tray.

6. Beat the lactose-free cream until thick.

7. To assemble the pavlova crunch, using your hands, break the pavlova up into large chunks and arrange on a serving dish.

8. Pour over the whipped cream and arrange the mixed berries on top of the cream. Drizzle the passionfruit over the top and serve.

RICE PUDDING WITH BERRY COMPOTE

SERVES 4

½ cup (120g/4oz) medium grain rice
600ml (1¼pt) unsweetened
  almond milk
¾ cup water
50g (2oz) castor sugar
1 tsp vanilla essence (extract)
1 tsp cinnamon

BERRY COMPOTE

¼ cup strawberries (fresh or frozen),
  hulled and quartered
¾ cup raspberries (fresh or frozen)
1 tbsp castor sugar
1 tbsp lemon juice
1 tbsp water

Energy 992kJ/237 Calories, Protein 3.5g,
Total Fat 4.6g, Saturated Fat 0.4g,
Carbohydrate 44.4g, Sugars 21.9g, Dietary
fibre 2.6g, Calcium 123.5mg, Iron 0.5mg.

1. Wash the rice in a sieve under cold water and drain well.

2. Place the rice, almond milk, water, sugar, vanilla and cinnamon in a large saucepan over very low heat and cook, stirring every few minutes, for 45 minutes or until the rice is cooked through and the mixture is thick and creamy.

3. Meanwhile, to make the compote, place the strawberries, raspberries, sugar, lemon juice and water in a small saucepan and bring to the boil. Reduce heat and simmer 3–5 minutes or until the fruit has softened. Remove from heat and set aside.

4. To serve, divide the rice pudding between serving bowls and top it with the berry compote.

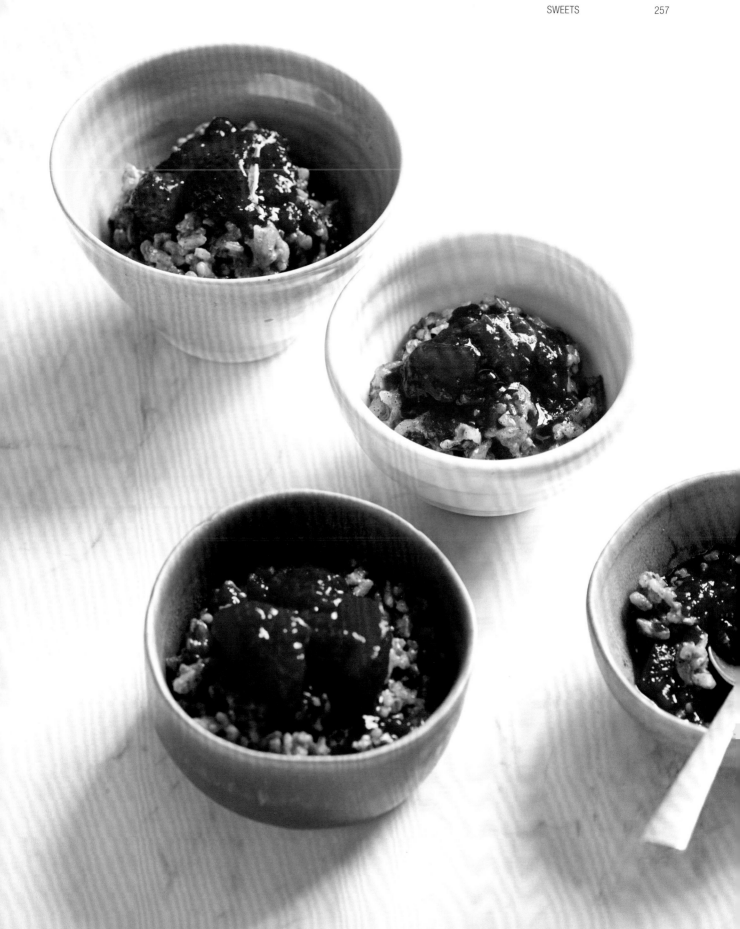

ORANGE AND POLENTA CAKE

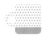

SERVES 10

200g (7oz) butter, softened
200g (7oz) demerara sugar
3 large eggs
1 tsp vanilla essence (extract)
200g (7oz) ground almonds
100g (3½oz) polenta
2 oranges, zested and juiced
1 tsp orange blossom water
1 tsp baking powder

SYRUP

5 cardamom pods
250ml (9fl oz) freshly squeezed
  orange juice
30ml (1fl oz) orange blossom water
125g (4½oz) raw castor sugar

Energy 1915kJ/458 Calories, Protein 7.3g,
Total Fat 29.0g, Saturated Fat 11.8g,
Carbohydrate 41.7g, Sugars 35.1g, Dietary
fibre 2.6g, Calcium 60.7mg, Iron 1.0mg.

1. Preheat the oven to 160°C/320°F. Grease a 20cm (8 inch) springform tin and line with baking paper.

2. Combine the butter and sugar in a large bowl and beat until light and creamy. Beat in the eggs, one at a time, then add the vanilla essence.

3. In a small bowl, mix together the ground almonds, polenta, orange zest, orange blossom water and baking powder. Blend these ingredients into the cake batter.

4. Pour the cake mixture into the prepared tin and bake for 40 to 50 minutes, or until the surface is lightly browned and the cake is detaching slightly from the sides of the tin.

5. Remove the tin from the oven and leave to cool for 10 minutes. Turn the cake out onto a plate. Take care as the cake is fragile.

6. To make the syrup, crush the cardamom pods and add them to a saucepan along with all the other remaining ingredients. Simmer over medium-low heat for approximately 10 minutes, or until the liquid has reduced and starts to thicken. Remove the cardamom pods (discard) and set aside to cool.

7. Puncture the cake several times with a skewer. Brush the cake generously with the syrup. Serve with a low lactose cream or yoghurt and an extra drizzle of syrup if desired.

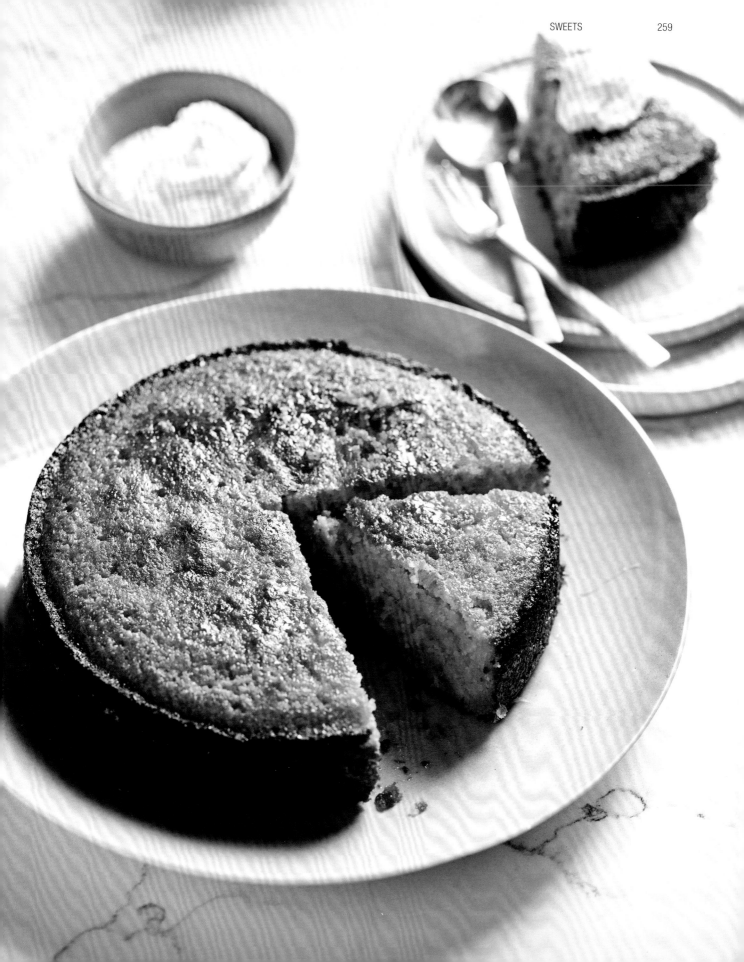

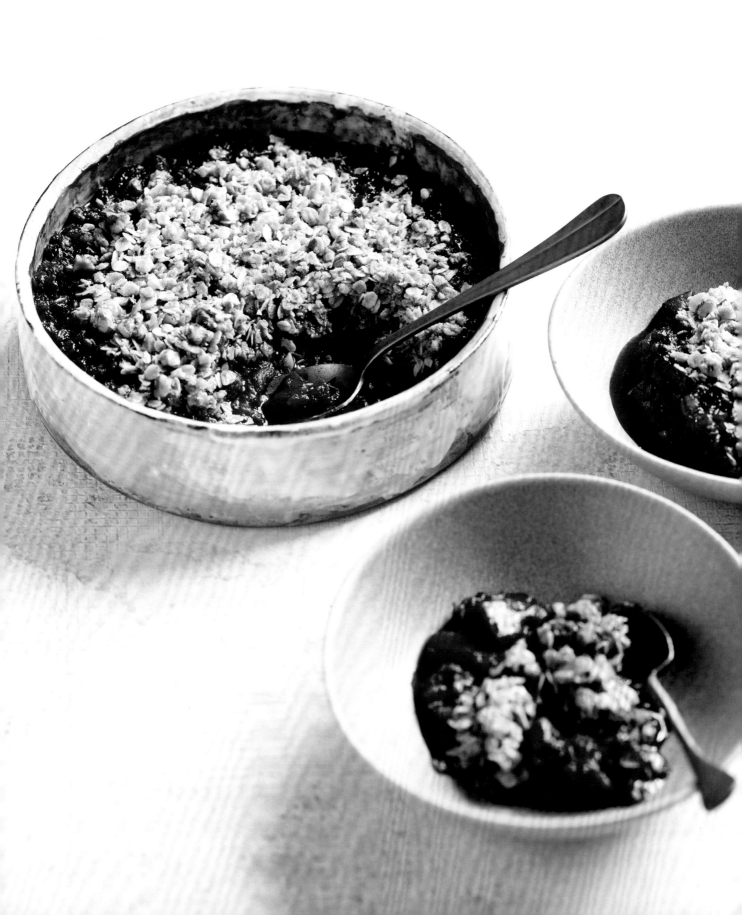

RASPBERRY AND RHUBARB CRUMBLE

SERVES 6

700g (1lb 5oz) trimmed rhubarb
    stems, cut into 2.5cm (1 inch)
    lengths
1 lemon, zested
1 tbsp water
½ cup castor sugar
100g (3½oz) raspberries (fresh
    or frozen)

CRUMBLE

1 cup (100g/3½oz) rolled oats
1 cup (125g/4½oz) gluten-free flour
1 tsp cinnamon
½ tsp salt
½ cup brown sugar
½ cup walnuts, roughly chopped
½ cup (100g/3½oz) coconut oil

Energy 1960kJ/468 Calories, Protein 6.3g,
Total Fat 26.2g, Saturated Fat 14.7g,
Carbohydrate 51.4g, Sugars 33.5g, Dietary
fibre 6.2g, Calcium 78.4mg, Iron 1.7mg.

1. Preheat the oven to 180°C/350°F.

2. Add the rhubarb, lemon zest, water and castor sugar to a saucepan and simmer over medium heat for 10 minutes or until the rhubarb starts to soften and collapse. When the rhubarb is almost ready, add the raspberries and cook for two minutes or until well combined and softened. Remove from the heat and set aside.

3. To make the crumble, place the oats, gluten-free flour, cinnamon, salt, walnuts and brown sugar into a large bowl and stir to combine.

4. Add the melted coconut oil to the crumble mixture and mix together to form a chunky crumble.

5. Transfer the rhubarb mixture to a baking dish set over a baking tray to catch any cooking juices. Top with crumble, then bake for 30 minutes or until golden. Serve warm or hot.

MEAL PLANNERS

This section elaborates on the FODMAP stacking menu suggestions. The purpose of this section is to provide ideas on how the recipes can be combined and adapted.

MAINS	• PANCAKES	• BREAKFAST MUFFINS • MUSHROOM RISOTTO • SPINACH AND PANEER CURRY • BAKED FISH WITH GINGER, SESAME AND SOY • THAI CRISPY FISH • HERBY ROAST CHICKEN • KUNG PAO CHICKEN • TANDOORI CHICKEN • CHINESE BRAISED BEEF NOODLES • NASI GORENG • FRENCH LAMB SHANKS	• CARROT AND ZUCCHINI FRITTERS WITH POACHED EGGS • SPINACH, FETTA AND PINE NUT OMELETTE • GREENS BREAKFAST PIE • PAELLA • PERSIAN PILAF • KOREAN GLASS NOODLE STIR-FRY • VEGGIE BURGER • PAD THAI • MIDDLE EASTERN FISH WITH TAHINI SAUCE • SALMON POKE BOWL • CHICKEN TACOS • CHICKEN CACCIATORE • SUMAC ROASTED CHICKEN WITH POLENTA • INDIAN CHICKEN CURRY WITH COCONUT MILK • LASAGNE • LAMB ROGAN JOSH • BEEF BURGUNDY

- SHAKSHOUKA
- SCRAMBLED TOFU
- VEGAN FRENCH TOAST
- WALNUT, SEED AND COCONUT GRANOLA
- BANANA BREAD SMOOTHIE
- GREEN SMOOTHIE
- MILLET SALAD WITH PESTO YOGHURT DRESSING
- INDIAN RICE WITH VEGETABLES
- MISO CHICKEN RAMEN
- INDIAN CHANNA DAHL
- SWEET POTATO OKONOMIYAKI
- STUFFED CAPSICUMS
- FISH WITH LEMON, BASIL AND GREEN BEANS
- THAI BEEF SALAD
- JAPANESE BEEF CURRY
- MIDDLE EASTERN BAKED KOFTAS
- SWEET AND SOUR PORK

- CINNAMON CHOC CHIP OVERNIGHT OATS
- STRAWBERRY AND WALNUT OVERNIGHT OATS
- CACAO SMOOTHIE BOWL
- QUINOA BUDDHA BOWL
- PUTTANESCA
- TERIYAKI TOFU BOWL
- GADO GADO
- SALMON AND EDAMAME SOBA NOODLE STIR-FRY
- THAI GREEN CHICKEN CURRY
- CHICKEN PROVENÇALE
- SPAGHETTI BOLOGNESE
- MALAYSIAN BEEF CURRY

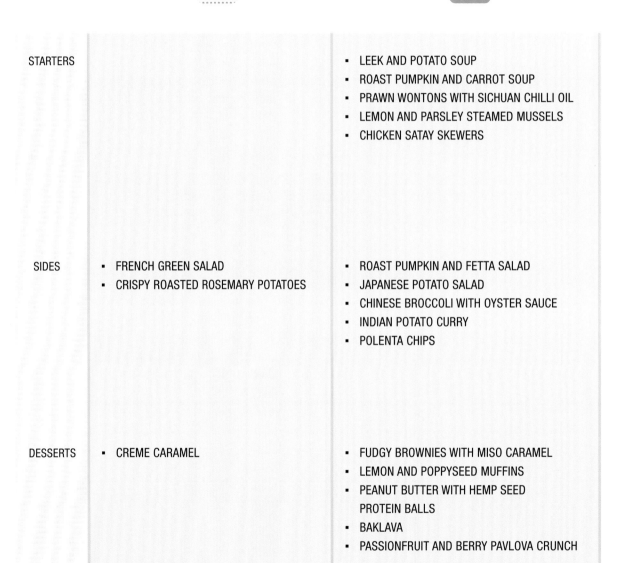

STARTERS		• LEEK AND POTATO SOUP
		• ROAST PUMPKIN AND CARROT SOUP
		• PRAWN WONTONS WITH SICHUAN CHILLI OIL
		• LEMON AND PARSLEY STEAMED MUSSELS
		• CHICKEN SATAY SKEWERS
SIDES	• FRENCH GREEN SALAD	• ROAST PUMPKIN AND FETTA SALAD
	• CRISPY ROASTED ROSEMARY POTATOES	• JAPANESE POTATO SALAD
		• CHINESE BROCCOLI WITH OYSTER SAUCE
		• INDIAN POTATO CURRY
		• POLENTA CHIPS
DESSERTS	• CREME CARAMEL	• FUDGY BROWNIES WITH MISO CARAMEL
		• LEMON AND POPPYSEED MUFFINS
		• PEANUT BUTTER WITH HEMP SEED PROTEIN BALLS
		• BAKLAVA
		• PASSIONFRUIT AND BERRY PAVLOVA CRUNCH

- HOT AND SOUR SOUP
- MISO SOUP
- PRAWN PHO
- TOM YUM SOUP
- THAI FISH CAKES
- CHICKEN YAKITORI

- GREEN FALAFELS
- VIETNAMESE RICE PAPER ROLLS
- SAN CHOY BAU
- SPICY TUNA SUSHI

- GREEN PAPAYA SALAD
- SPICY THAI CUCUMBER SALAD
- TABOULI
- MISO GLAZED EGGPLANT
- CHINESE STYLE EGGPLANT
- LEMON AND PARSLEY GREEN
  BEANS

- FATTOUSH SALAD
- CAPRESE SALAD
- SALAD NICOISE
- ROASTED VEGETABLES
  WITH BALSAMIC
- SLOW-ROASTED TRUSS TOMATOES
- THAI VEGETABLE STIR-FRY
- THAI GREEN BEANS

- RATATOUILLE

- TAHINI CHOCOLATE CHIP COOKIES
- OAT AND SEED BISCUITS
- RICE PUDDING WITH
  BERRY COMPOTE
- RASPBERRY AND
  RHUBARB CRUMBLE

INTERNATIONAL FLAVOURS
SERVING SUGGESTIONS

This table will help you to combine recipes to create meal plans. The recipes are arranged in their various international categories as a guide to which recipes complement each other. The low FODMAP stack cup rating per serve of each dish is also provided.

Plan your meal using the Monash low FODMAP stack cup.

INDIAN FLAVOURS

MAIN DISH

LAMB ROGAN JOSH
PAGE 212

INDIAN CHANNA DAHL
PAGE 138   (Ve)

SIDE DISH

INDIAN POTATO CURRY
PAGE 77   (Ve)

SPINACH AND PANEER
CURRY PAGE 152   (V)

INDIAN CORIANDER AND
MINT RAITA PAGE 233   (V)

THAI FLAVOURS

MAIN DISH			SIDE DISH		

MAIN DISH

THAI FISH CAKES
PAGE 172

PAD THAI
PAGE 143

THAI BEEF SALAD
PAGE 203

THAI GREEN CHICKEN
CURRY PAGE 182

THAI CRISPY FISH
PAGE 174

SIDE DISH

SPICY THAI
CUCUMBER SALAD
PAGE 61

GREEN PAPAYA SALAD
PAGE 54

TOM YUM SOUP
PAGE 125

THAI GREEN BEANS
PAGE 89

THAI VEGETABLE
STIR-FRY PAGE 84

CHINESE FLAVOURS

MAIN DISH

BAKED FISH WITH
GINGER SESAME
AND SOY PAGE 168

CHINESE BRAISED BEEF
NOODLES PAGE 220

KUNG PAO CHICKEN
PAGE 189

PRAWN WONTONS WITH
SICHUAN CHILLI OIL
PAGE 160

SWEET AND SOUR PORK
PAGE 217

SIDE DISH

CHINESE BROCCOLI
WITH OYSTER SAUCE
PAGE 72

HOT AND SOUR SOUP
PAGE 113

CHINESE STYLE
EGGPLANT PAGE 78

SAN CHOY BAU
PAGE 144

ITALIAN FLAVOURS

MAIN DISH

LASAGNE

FISH WITH LEMON, BASIL
AND GREEN BEANS

SPAGHETT BOLOGNESE

MUSHROOM RISOTTO

PUTTANESCA

SIDE DISH

CRISPY ROSEMARY
ROASTED POTATOES

CAPRESE SALAD

SLOW-ROASTED TRUSS
TOMATOES

'GARLIC' AIOLI

ROASTED GREEN AND
RED CAPSICUM

POLENTA CHIPS

JAPANESE FLAVOURS

MAIN DISH

CHICKEN YAKITORI
PAGE 195

MISO CHICKEN RAMEN
PAGE 120

JAPANESE BEEF CURRY
PAGE 205

TUNA SUSHI
PAGE 171

TERIYAKI TOFU BOWL
PAGE 137

SALMON AND SOBA
NOODLE STIR-FRY
PAGE 157

SIDE DISH

JAPANESE POTATO
SALAD PAGE 58

MISO GLAZED
EGGPLANT PAGE 71

MISO SOUP
PAGE 114

SWEET POTATO
OKONOMIYAKI
PAGE 146

MIDDLE EASTERN FLAVOURS

MAIN DISH		SIDE DISH	

SUMAC ROASTED CHICKEN WITH POLENTA
PAGE 190

TABOULI SALAD
PAGE 64

MIDDLE EASTERN BAKED KOFTAS PAGE 211

PERSIAN PILAF
PAGE 106

MIDDLE EASTERN FISH WITH TAHINI SAUCE
PAGE 158

FATTOUSH SALAD
PAGE 48

GREEN FALAFELS
PAGE 132 (Ve)

SHAKSHUKA
PAGE 23

STUFFED CAPSICUMS
PAGE 151

ASIAN FLAVOURS

MAIN DISH		SIDE DISH	

CHICKEN SATAY SKEWERS PAGE 180

KOREAN GLASS NOODLES STIR-FRY
PAGE 135

VIETNAMESE RICE PAPER ROLLS PAGE 129

NASI GORENG
PAGE 103

PRAWN PHO
PAGE 117

GADO GADO
PAGE 149

FRENCH FLAVOURS

MAIN DISH	SIDE DISH

LEMON AND PARSLEY
STEAMED MUSSELS
PAGE 166

LEEK AND POTATO SOUP
PAGE 119

BEEF BURGUNDY
PAGE 222

RATATOUILLE
PAGE 131

FRENCH LAMB SHANKS
PAGE 214

LEMON PARSLEY
GREENS BEANS PAGE 87

CHICKEN PROVENÇALE
PAGE 198

FRENCH GREEN SALAD
PAGE 51

SALAD NICOISE
PAGE 63

ROASTED VEGETABLES
WITH BALSAMIC
PAGE 68

SPINACH, FETTA AND
PINE NUT OMELETTE
PAGE 26

FRENCH DRESSING
PAGE 228

NUTRIENT INFOGRAPHICS

A low FODMAP diet is a restrictive diet that without careful planning can compromise intake of a number of key nutrients. Nutrients at particular risk include protein, iron, calcium and fibre. These nutrients are important at all life stages and for a number of key bodily functions.

For example, protein is needed to help your cells to grow and repair properly; iron is needed to transport oxygen in the blood; calcium is needed to build and maintain strong bones; and fibre is needed for a healthy digestive system. Working with an experienced dietitian can help to ensure that you follow the 3 step FODMAP diet properly, while also optimising your nutritional intake.

This cookbook is designed to help you to follow a healthy, low FODMAP diet. The recipes are not only delicious and low in FODMAPs, but they're also highly nutritious.

To help you to identify recipes that are good sources of key nutrients (protein, iron, calcium and fibre) we have included icons on each recipe. The following charts summarise this information and allow you to compare the nutrient content of different recipes.

For example, you might notice that while there are some vegetarian and vegan dishes which are good sources of iron and protein, meat dishes are the best source of these nutrients.

HIGH IN PROTEIN

■ animal-based ▫ vegetarian

Sumac roasted chicken with polenta	Page 190
Chinese braised beef noodles	Page 220
Indian chicken curry with coconut milk	Page 192
Paella	Page 92
Salmon and soba noodle stir-fry	Page 157
Baked fish with ginger sesame and soy	Page 168
Miso chicken ramen	Page 120
French lamb shanks	Page 214
Middle eastern fish with tahini sauce	Page 158
Sweet and sour pork	Page 217
Middle Eastern baked koftas	Page 211
Beef Burgundy	Page 222
Nasi goreng	Page 103
Salad Nicoise	Page 63
Kung pao chicken	Page 189
Japanese beef curry	Page 205
Thai beef salad	Page 203
Fish with lemon, basil and green beans	Page 163
Herby roast chicken	Page 179
Salmon poke bowl	Page 165
Lemon and parsley steamed mussels	Page 166
Chicken yakitori	Page 195
Spaghetti bolognaise	Page 206
Thai crispy fish	Page 174
Chicken provecale	Page 198
Lamb rogan josh	Page 212
Thai fish cakes	Page 172
Lasagne	Page 209
Teriyaki tofu bowls	Page 137
Malaysian beef curry	Page 219
Prawn pho	Page 117
Tandoori chicken	Page 197
Chicken cacciatore	Page 186
Tuna sushi	Page 171
Chicken tacos	Page 185
Spinach, fetta and pine nut omelette	Page 26
Tom yum soup	Page 125
Gado gado	Page 149
Prawn wontons with sichuan chilli oil	Page 160
Thai green chicken curry	Page 182
Scrambled tofu	Page 29
Quinoa Buddha bowl	Page 99
Chicken satay skewers	Page 180
Vegan French toast	Page 30
Hot and sour soup	Page 113
Vietnamese rice paper rolls	Page 129
Cinnamon choc chips overnight oats	Page 36
Mushroom risotto	Page 94
Pad Thai	Page 143
Japanese potato salad	Page 58
Strawberry and walnut overnight oats	Page 36
Korean glass noodle stir-fry	Page 135
Millet salad with pesto yoghurt dressing	Page 97
Cacao smoothie bowl	Page 41
Shakshouka	Page 23
San choy bau	Page 144
Puttanesca	Page 105
Stuffed capsicums	Page 151
Greens breakfast pie	Page 44
Sweet potato okonomiyaki	Page 146
Green smoothie	Page 42
Spinach and paneer curry	Page 152
Green falafels	Page 132
Carrot and zucchini fritters with poached eggs	Page 24
Veggie burgers	Page 140
Miso soup	Page 114

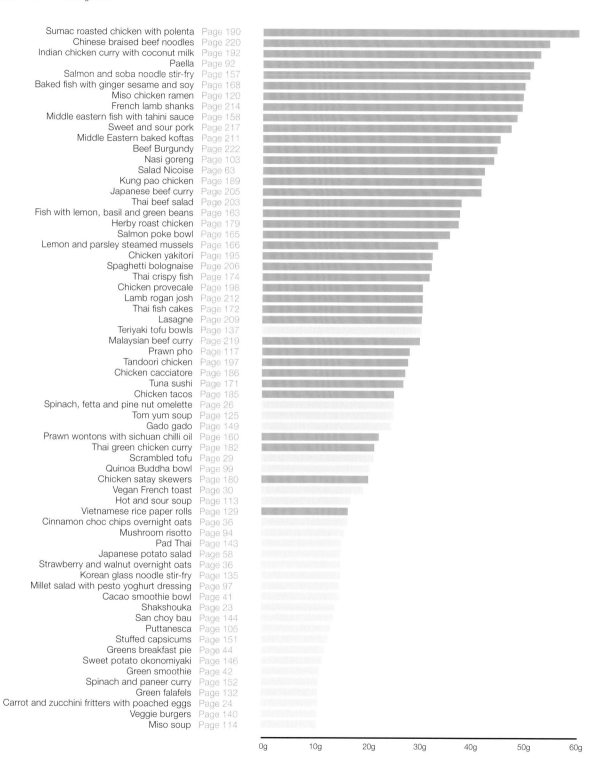

0g   10g   20g   30g   40g   50g   60g

HIGH IN CALCIUM

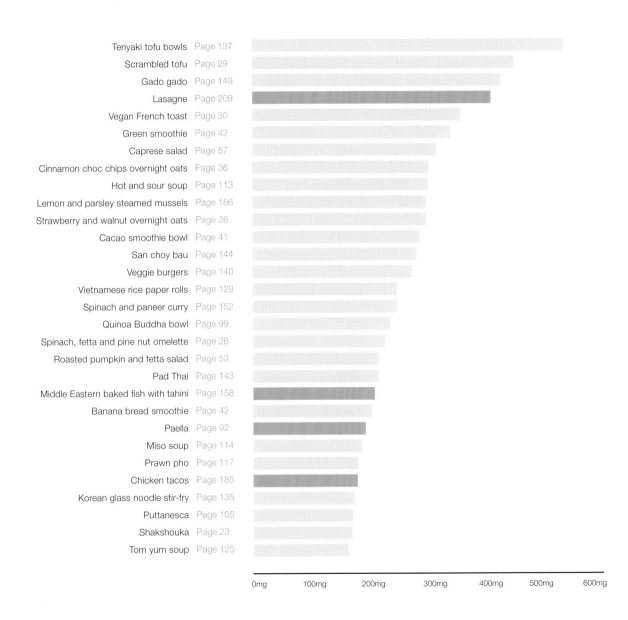

animal-based   vegetarian

Teriyaki tofu bowls	Page 137
Scrambled tofu	Page 29
Gado gado	Page 149
Lasagne	Page 209
Vegan French toast	Page 30
Green smoothie	Page 42
Caprese salad	Page 57
Cinnamon choc chips overnight oats	Page 36
Hot and sour soup	Page 113
Lemon and parsley steamed mussels	Page 166
Strawberry and walnut overnight oats	Page 36
Cacao smoothie bowl	Page 41
San choy bau	Page 144
Veggie burgers	Page 140
Vietnamese rice paper rolls	Page 129
Spinach and paneer curry	Page 152
Quinoa Buddha bowl	Page 99
Spinach, fetta and pine nut omelette	Page 26
Roasted pumpkin and fetta salad	Page 53
Pad Thai	Page 143
Middle Eastern baked fish with tahini	Page 158
Banana bread smoothie	Page 42
Paella	Page 92
Miso soup	Page 114
Prawn pho	Page 117
Chicken tacos	Page 185
Korean glass noodle stir-fry	Page 135
Puttanesca	Page 105
Shakshouka	Page 23
Tom yum soup	Page 125

0mg   100mg   200mg   300mg   400mg   500mg   600mg

HIGH IN IRON

■ animal-based   ▢ vegetarian

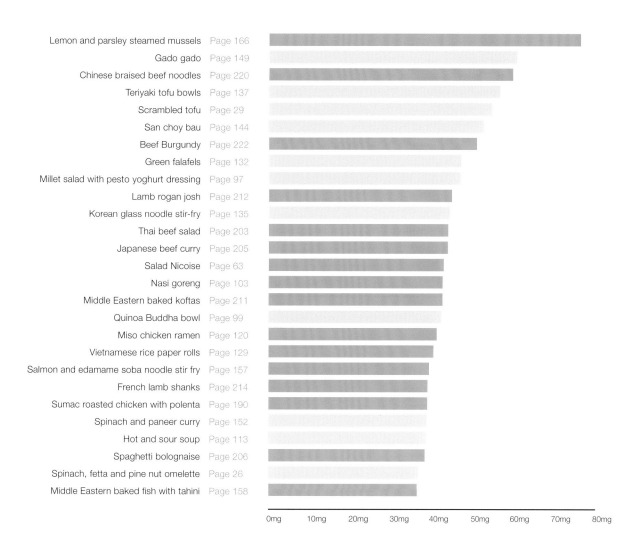

Lemon and parsley steamed mussels	Page 166
Gado gado	Page 149
Chinese braised beef noodles	Page 220
Teriyaki tofu bowls	Page 137
Scrambled tofu	Page 29
San choy bau	Page 144
Beef Burgundy	Page 222
Green falafels	Page 132
Millet salad with pesto yoghurt dressing	Page 97
Lamb rogan josh	Page 212
Korean glass noodle stir-fry	Page 135
Thai beef salad	Page 203
Japanese beef curry	Page 205
Salad Nicoise	Page 63
Nasi goreng	Page 103
Middle Eastern baked koftas	Page 211
Quinoa Buddha bowl	Page 99
Miso chicken ramen	Page 120
Vietnamese rice paper rolls	Page 129
Salmon and edamame soba noodle stir fry	Page 157
French lamb shanks	Page 214
Sumac roasted chicken with polenta	Page 190
Spinach and paneer curry	Page 152
Hot and sour soup	Page 113
Spaghetti bolognaise	Page 206
Spinach, fetta and pine nut omelette	Page 26
Middle Eastern baked fish with tahini	Page 158

0mg   10mg   20mg   30mg   40mg   50mg   60mg   70mg   80mg

HIGH IN FIBRE

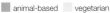

■ animal-based ■ vegetarian

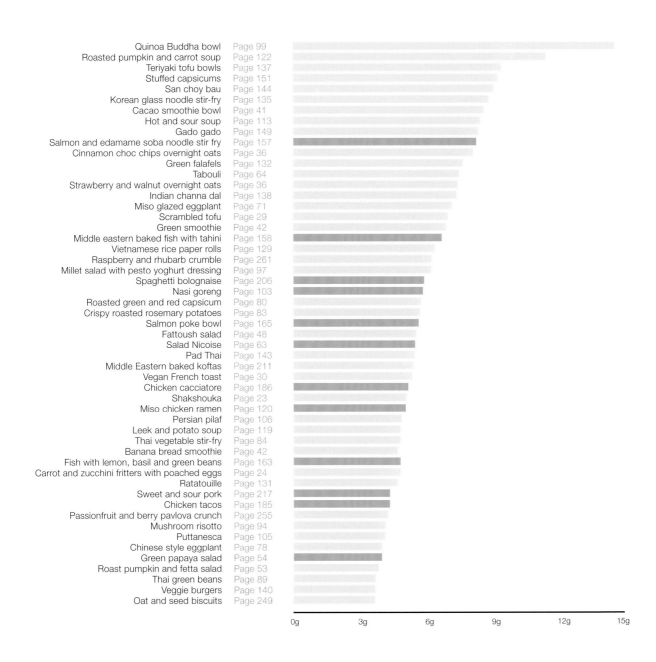

Quinoa Buddha bowl	Page 99
Roasted pumpkin and carrot soup	Page 122
Teriyaki tofu bowls	Page 137
Stuffed capsicums	Page 151
San choy bau	Page 144
Korean glass noodle stir-fry	Page 135
Cacao smoothie bowl	Page 41
Hot and sour soup	Page 113
Gado gado	Page 149
Salmon and edamame soba noodle stir fry	Page 157
Cinnamon choc chips overnight oats	Page 36
Green falafels	Page 132
Tabouli	Page 64
Strawberry and walnut overnight oats	Page 36
Indian channa dal	Page 138
Miso glazed eggplant	Page 71
Scrambled tofu	Page 29
Green smoothie	Page 42
Middle eastern baked fish with tahini	Page 158
Vietnamese rice paper rolls	Page 129
Raspberry and rhubarb crumble	Page 261
Millet salad with pesto yoghurt dressing	Page 97
Spaghetti bolognaise	Page 206
Nasi goreng	Page 103
Roasted green and red capsicum	Page 80
Crispy roasted rosemary potatoes	Page 83
Salmon poke bowl	Page 165
Fattoush salad	Page 48
Salad Nicoise	Page 63
Pad Thai	Page 143
Middle Eastern baked koftas	Page 211
Vegan French toast	Page 30
Chicken cacciatore	Page 186
Shakshouka	Page 23
Miso chicken ramen	Page 120
Persian pilaf	Page 106
Leek and potato soup	Page 119
Thai vegetable stir-fry	Page 84
Banana bread smoothie	Page 42
Fish with lemon, basil and green beans	Page 163
Carrot and zucchini fritters with poached eggs	Page 24
Ratatouille	Page 131
Sweet and sour pork	Page 217
Chicken tacos	Page 185
Passionfruit and berry pavlova crunch	Page 255
Mushroom risotto	Page 94
Puttanesca	Page 105
Chinese style eggplant	Page 78
Green papaya salad	Page 54
Roast pumpkin and fetta salad	Page 53
Thai green beans	Page 89
Veggie burgers	Page 140
Oat and seed biscuits	Page 249

0g   3g   6g   9g   12g   15g

FODMAP STACK CUP RATINGS FOR VEGETABLE AND FRUIT COMBINATIONS

The following foods are simple combinations of vegetables and fruits that are low in FODMAPs with the FODMAP stack cup rating.

Use this information to make your own recipes. For the vegetable combinations just add a good source of protein and a low FODMAP grain to make a complete meal.

VEGETABLE COMBINATIONS

THAI

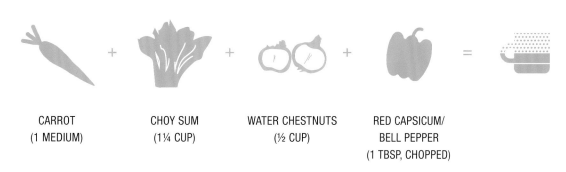

CARROT	CHOY SUM	WATER CHESTNUTS	RED CAPSICUM/
(1 MEDIUM)	(1¼ CUP)	(½ CUP)	BELL PEPPER
			(1 TBSP, CHOPPED)

JAPANESE

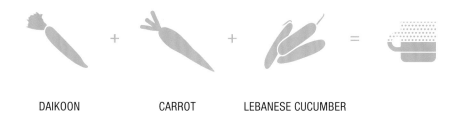

DAIKOON   CARROT   LEBANESE CUCUMBER
(½ CUP, CHOPPED)   (1 MEDIUM)   (½ CUP, CHOPPED)

INDIAN

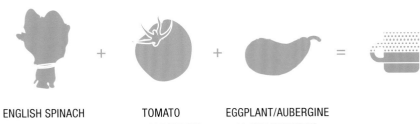

ENGLISH SPINACH
(1½ CUP, CHOPPED)

TOMATO
(COMMON/TRUSS)
(½, SMALL)

EGGPLANT/AUBERGINE
(1 CUP, CHOPPED)

MIDDLE EASTERN

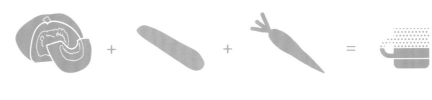

JAPANESE PUMPKIN
(½ CUP, CHOPPED)

ZUCCHINI/COURGETTE
(½ CUP, CHOPPED)

CARROT
(½ MEDIUM)

AUSTRALIAN

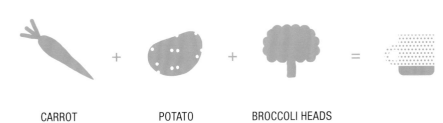

CARROT
(1 MEDIUM)

POTATO
(½ MEDIUM)

BROCCOLI HEADS
(½ CUP, CHOPPED)

USA

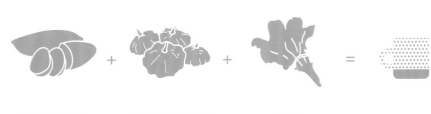

SWEET POTATO
(¼ CUP, CHOPPED)

PATTYPAN SQUASH
(1 MEDIUM)

KALE
(½ CUP, CHOPPED)

GERMAN

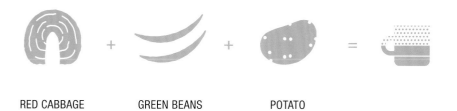

RED CABBAGE
(½ CUP, CHOPPED)

GREEN BEANS
(7 BEANS)

POTATO
(½ MEDIUM)

TEX-MEX

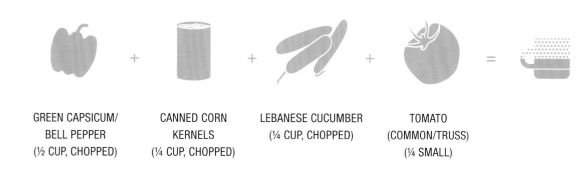

GREEN CAPSICUM/
BELL PEPPER
(½ CUP, CHOPPED)

CANNED CORN
KERNELS
(¼ CUP, CHOPPED)

LEBANESE CUCUMBER
(¼ CUP, CHOPPED)

TOMATO
(COMMON/TRUSS)
(¼ SMALL)

ITALIAN

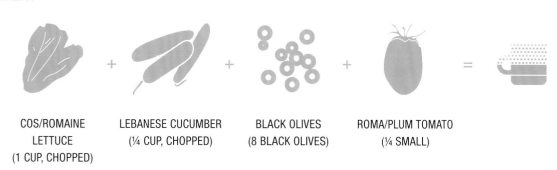

COS/ROMAINE
LETTUCE
(1 CUP, CHOPPED)

LEBANESE CUCUMBER
(¼ CUP, CHOPPED)

BLACK OLIVES
(8 BLACK OLIVES)

ROMA/PLUM TOMATO
(¼ SMALL)

VEGAN

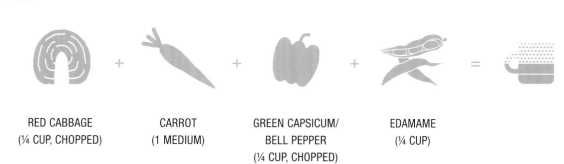

RED CABBAGE
(¼ CUP, CHOPPED)

CARROT
(1 MEDIUM)

GREEN CAPSICUM/
BELL PEPPER
(¼ CUP, CHOPPED)

EDAMAME
(¼ CUP)

FRUIT COMBINATIONS

FRUIT COMBINATION 1

 + + =

RAW MANDARIN/
CLEMENTINE
(¼ MEDIUM)

FIRM BANANA
(½ MEDIUM)

PEELED GREEN KIWI
FRUIT
(½ MEDIUM)

FRUIT COMBINATION 2

 + + =

DRAGONFRUIT
(½ MEDIUM)

RASPBERRIES
(15 BERRIES)

YELLOW PAPAYA
(½ CUP, CHOPPED)

FRUIT COMBINATION 3

 + + =

STARFRUIT/
CARAMBOLA
(½ MEDIUM)

CANTALOUPE/
ROCKMELON
(½ CUP, CHOPPED)

PINEAPPLE
(½ CUP, CHOPPED)

FRUIT COMBINATION 4

 + + =

PASSIONFRUIT
(1 MEDIUM)

NAVEL ORANGE
(¼ MEDIUM)

BLUEBERRIES
(¼ CUP)

FRUIT COMBINATION 5

 + + 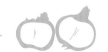 + =

AÇAI POWDER
(1 TEASPOON)

HONEYDEW MELON
(¼ CUP, CHOPPED)

WATER CHESTNUTS
(½ CUP)

FRESH/FROZEN
CRANBERRIES
(½ CUP)

BIBLIOGRAPHY

1. Halmos EP, Power VA, Shepherd SJ, Gibson PR, Muir JG. A diet low in FODMAPs reduces symptoms of irritable bowel syndrome. Gastroenterology. 2014;146(1):67-75. e5.

2. Biesiekierski JR, Peters SL, Newnham ED, Rosella O, Muir JG, Gibson PR. No effects of gluten in patients with self-reported non-celiac gluten sensitivity after dietary reduction of fermentable, poorly absorbed, short-chain carbohydrates. Gastroenterology. 2013;145(2):320-8. e1-3.

3. Peters SL, Yao CK, Philpott H, Yelland GW, Muir JG, Gibson PR. Randomised clinical trial: the efficacy of gut-directed hypnotherapy is similar to that of the low FODMAP diet for the treatment of irritable bowel syndrome. Alimentary Pharmacology and Therapeutics. 2016;44(5):447-59.

4. Ong DK, Mitchell SB, Barrett JS, Shepherd SJ, Irving PM, Biesiekierski JR, Smith S, Gibson PR, Muir JG. Manipulation of dietary short chain carbohydrates alters the pattern of gas production and genesis of symptoms in irritable bowel syndrome. Journal of Gastroenterology and Hepatology. 2010;25(8):1366-73.

5. Barrett JS, R. B. Gearry RB, J. G. Muir JG, P. M. Irving PM, R. Rose R, O. Rosella O, Haines ML, Shepherd SJ, Gibson PR. Dietary poorly absorbed, short-chain carbohydrates increase delivery of water and fermentable substrates to the proximal colon. Alimentary Pharmacology and Therapeutics. 2010;31, 874–882.

6. Muir JG, Shepherd SJ, Rosella O, Rose R, Barrett JS, Gibson PR. Fructan and free fructose content of common Australian vegetables and fruit. Journal of Agricultural and Food Chemistry. 2007;55(16):6619-27.

7. Muir JG, Rose R, Rosella O, Liels K, Barrett JS, Shepherd SJ, Gibson PR. Measurement of short-chain carbohydrates in common Australian vegetables and fruits by high-performance liquid chromatography (HPLC). Journal of Agricultural and Food Chemistry. 2009;57(2):554-65.

8. Biesiekierski JR, Rosella O, Rose R, Liels K, Barrett SJ, Shepherd SJ, Gibson PR, Muir JG. Quantification of fructans, galacto-oligosacharides and other short-chain carbohydrates in processed grains and cereals. Journal of Human Nutrition and Dietetics. 2011;24(2):154-76.

9. Gibson PR, Shepherd SJ. Personal view: food for thought-western lifestyle and susceptibility to Crohn's disease. The FODMAP hypothesis. Alimentary Pharmacology and Therapeutics. 2005;21(12):1399-409.

10. Tuck C, Ly E, Bogatyrev A, Costetsou I, Gibson P, Barrett J, Muir JG. Fermentable short chain carbohydrate (FODMAP) content of common plant-based foods and processed foods suitable for vegetarian- and vegan-based eating patterns. Journal of Human Nutrition and Dietetics. 2018;31(3):422-35.

11. Varney J, Barrett J, Scarlata K, Catsos P, Gibson PR, Muir JG. FODMAPs: food composition, defining cutoff values and international application. Journal of Gastroenterology and Hepatology 2017; 32 (Suppl. 1): 53–61.

12. Staudacher HM, Kurien M, Whelan K. Nutritional implications of dietary interventions for managing gastrointestinal disorders. Current Opinion in Gastroenteroly. 2018;34(2):105-11.

13. Nutrition, Health and Related Claims Standard (Standard 1.2.7) 2016. Australia New Zealand Food Standards Code (the Food Standards Code). Available at https://www.legislation.gov.au/Details/F2016C00082

14. National Health and Medical Research Council, Australian Government Department of Health and Ageing, New Zealand Ministry of Health. Nutrient Reference Values for Australia and New Zealand. Canberra: National Health and Medical Research Council; 2006, updated 2017. Available at https://www.nhmrc.gov.au/about-us/publications

15. Food Standards Australia New Zealand (2022). Australian Food Composition Database – Release 2. Canberra: FSANZ. Available at www.foodstandards.gov.au

16. National Health and Medical Research Council (2013) Australian Dietary Guidelines Summary. Canberra: National Health and Medical Research Council. Available at www.eatforhealth.gov.au/guidelines

INDEX

Z

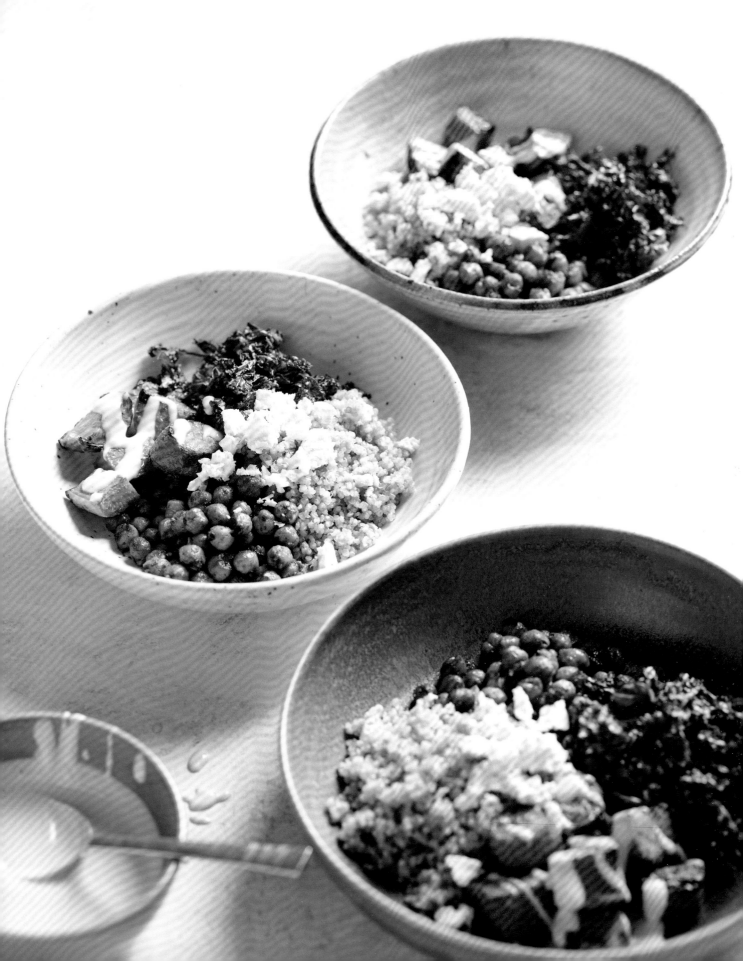

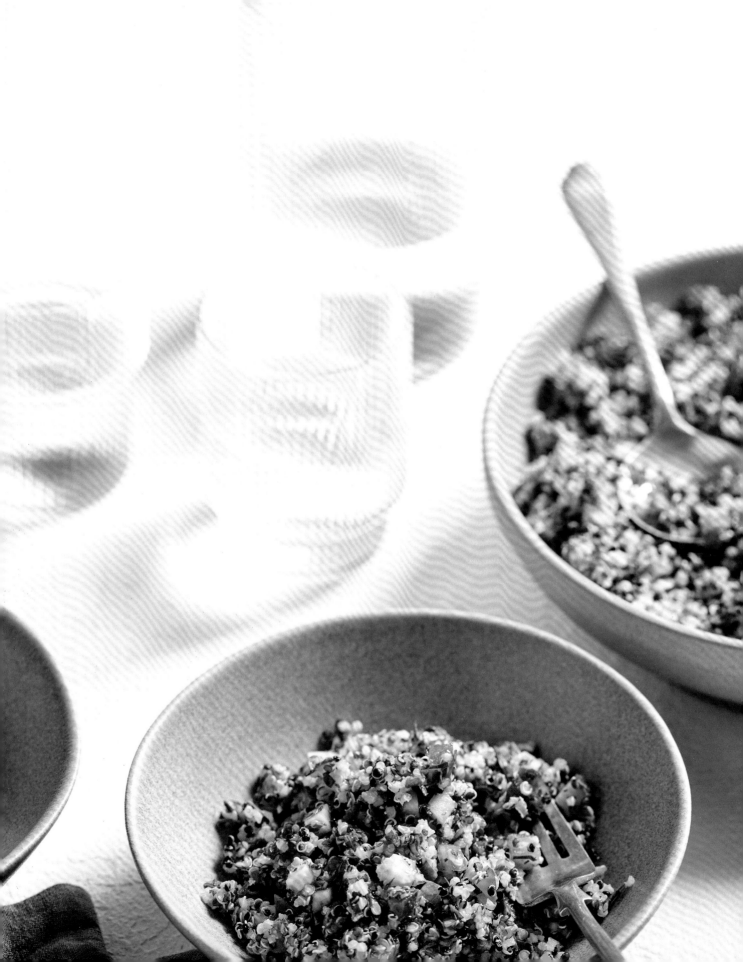

NOTES

MORE FROM US

OUR PATIENT COURSE

The expert team at Monash University has developed an online course to help IBS sufferers better understand their condition and how to safely follow a 3 step FODMAP diet.

The 5 module course is written with patients in mind, so there's no jargon or complex language. We simply teach you in plain English about everything you need to know to understand your condition and manage your symptoms using a FODMAP diet.

The course covers all the essential topics including:

- The importance of getting an accurate diagnosis of IBS

- What are FODMAPs and where are they found?

- How to implement Steps 1, 2 and 3 of the FODMAP diet

- Understanding whether your IBS symptoms are sensitive to FODMAPs

- What to do if your IBS symptoms do not improve on a low FODMAP diet

- Other therapies to help manage IBS symptoms.

Interactive elements are included all throughout the course, including videos, infographics, question-answer flip cards, sorting activities and interactive charts.

Because the course is delivered online, patients from all over the world can learn from the experts who pioneered FODMAP research at Monash University. You can also learn at your own pace, over 12 months and in the comfort of your own home. Go to our website monashfodmap.com for more information about the patient course.

THE MONASH FODMAP APP

The Monash University low FODMAP Diet App is your on-the-go guide to low FODMAP foods and the perfect companion to the Monash University Low FODMAP Cookbook. The App lists hundreds of foods that have been laboratory tested at Monash University and newly tested foods are frequently added. The App uses a simple traffic light rating system to indicate the overall rating of each food at a typical serving size - low (green), moderate (amber) or high (red) in FODMAPs, and displays which particular FODMAPs are present.

The Monash Low FODMAP Diet App also includes:

- Lists of food products from brands that have been tested and certified as low FODMAP

- Lists of meals and recipes that have been assessed and certified as low FODMAP

- A diary function that allows you to log your food intake and symptoms

- Instructions on completing the reintroduction phase

- A directory of thousands of dietitians from around the world who have undertaken the Monash Dietitian Training Course. These dietitians are trained in delivering a FODMAP diet to support patients with IBS.

The App is available from the App Store, Google Play or the Amazon App store. Revenue generated from App sales helps to support further FODMAP food analysis and research.

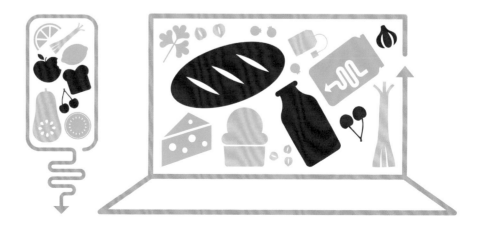

ACKNOWLEDGEMENTS

Monash University FODMAP Team

- Recipe Development: Jane Muir, Ally Heywood, Dakota Rhys-Jones, Jane Varney, Peter Gibson, Lyndal Collins, Jimmy Lee, Patricia Veitch

- Food analysis: Alex Bogatyrev and Elizabeth Ly

- Technical support: Balaji Nataragan

Project Editor — Clara Murphy

Design Consultation — Warren Taylor (Monash Art Design & Architecture)

Illustrations — Zach Beltsos-Russo

Food Photography and Styling — Mark Roper, Sarah Watson, Meryl Batlle and Lee Blaylock

Layout — Matthew Justice and Nils Bellarts

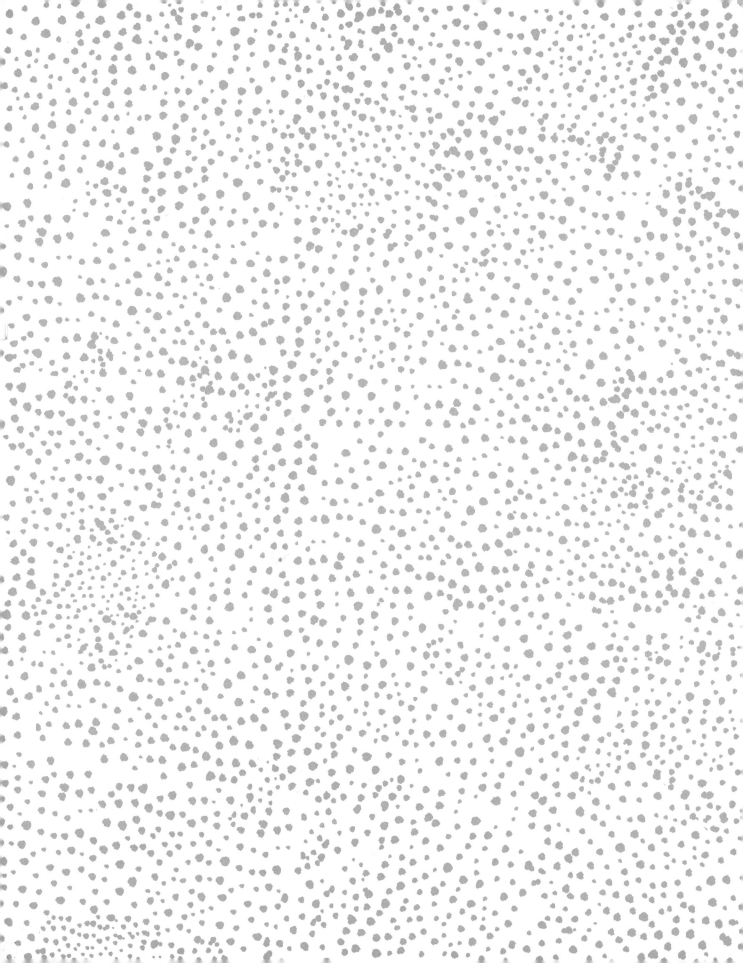